Safeguarding
the
Public Health

SAFEGUARDING
THE
PUBLIC HEALTH

NEWARK, 1895 – 1918

Stuart Galishoff

GREENWOOD PRESS

Westport, Connecticut • London, England

Library of Congress Cataloging in Publication Data

Galishoff, Stuart.
    Safeguarding the public health.

    Bibliography: p.
    Includes index.
    1. Hygiene, Public—New Jersey—Newark—History.
2. Public health administration—New Jersey—Newark—History. 3. Newark, N.J.—History. I. Title.
RA448.N73G34   362.1'09749'32   75-66
ISBN 0-8371-7956-4

Library of Congress Catalog Card Number: 75-66
ISBN 0-8371-7956-4

First published in 1975

Greenwood Press, a division of Williamhouse-Regency Inc.
51 Riverside Avenue, Westport, Connecticut 06880

Printed in the United States of America

To my parents

Contents

Tables

Charts

Preface

Public health has been defined as "the science and art of preventing
disease and promoting health through organized community activity."[1]
The pattern of disease in a community is dictated by circumstances of
time, place, and culture. To study fully a community's public health,
either in the past or the present, requires a grasp of many biological and
social forces. The researcher must be knowledgeable about the natural
history of disease, including such matters as the virulence of invading
microorganisms and the resistance of the host population. He must also
study socioeconomic conditions: housing, incomes, nutrition, working
conditions, family structure, and even folk medicine and local customs.

Ideally, then, a historical survey of a community's health should delve
deeply into all facets of its development. What did the poor eat? Were dairy
products available in the winter? Did the wage scale provide a standard of
living sufficient to maintain good health? How were houses constructed;
were they dry and were they screened and rodent-proof? As for infant and
maternal mortality, one would want to know the working conditions of
women, the quality of the milk supply, the prevalence of prostitution
and illegitimacy, the availability of competent medical care, and the child-
rearing practices of the various ethnic groups in the community. An
undertaking of such magnitude, however, embracing nearly all aspects of
life, is beyond anyone's resources. Having to keep the scope of his inquiry
within manageable limits, the public health historian must separate the
wheat from the chaff, deciding what was crucial to the community's
health and what was marginal. He must also try to see the events he narrates through the eyes of his subjects, and, of course, he can investigate
only those aspects of the past for which there are records.

In writing on public health in Newark for the years 1895-1918, I have
limited my investigation to those measures that best typify Newark's
response to the major health problems of that period. Consequently,

there is no discussion of early concern about drug addiction or of abortive smoke abatement campaigns. The primary focus of the study is the work of the Newark Board of Health and, more generally, the control of contagious diseases.

The 1890s are pivotal in Newark's public health history. In the decades following the Civil War, community leaders had largely ignored the health perils occasioned by the city's rapid growth and industrialization. Crowded tenements, hazardous industrial conditions, and a contaminated water supply had caused Newark to become one of the nation's most dangerous cities. Beginning about 1895, however, the city began to deal with its health problems and the death rate fell off sharply.

The 1890s also witnessed the advent of bacteriology. Until then, physicians had believed that epidemics resulted from the noxious vapors given off by decomposing filth. Thus the Newark Board of Health had attempted to prevent illness by keeping the streets clean and by urging on the public sanitary means of sewage and garbage disposal. For the most part, however, the board had failed, and the death rate remained high.

The establishment of a bacteriological laboratory in the Newark Department of Health in 1895 ushered in a new era in the city's health fortunes. The laboratory's success in combating diphtheria and other contagious diseases revitalized the department, which was given increased powers to safeguard the public health. Applying the knowledge uncovered by the germ theory of disease, the department in the years 1895-1918 effected a marked reduction in the city's death rate.

In 1916 Newark became a casualty of the nation's first great polio epidemic. Two years later "Spanish" influenza caused over 2,000 deaths in Newark. But these were parting salvos to a vanishing era in which pestilence had cast a long shadow over the city. After 1918 acute, communicable diseases ceased to be the great robbers of health and life they had been since the community's founding in 1666.

Two threads that run throughout this work may be noted: 1) increasing government assumption of responsibility for public health; and 2) the interaction of medicine and society. It seems likely that the pattern of events woven by these threads was much the same in other large American cities. Programs adopted in Newark to deal with the problems of tenement housing, industrial hygiene, and an impoverished milk supply were part of a national movement, and it would be surprising if successful innovations made in one city's public health services were not adopted in other communities. Still, it would be unwise to generalize about urban health reform on the basis of just one city's experiences. Inferences that might be drawn from Newark's public health history must be checked against the records of other cities. One final caveat: because of differences in location, ethnic composition, tradition, and economic development, each city's public health history is unique in certain regards. Comparing Newark with Boston,[2] for example, one finds that mosquitoes and water supply were serious problems in Newark but of minor consequence in Boston; conversely, maritime quarantine loomed large in Boston's history but mattered little in Newark.

Many persons helped to make this book possible. I wish to thank the staffs of the Newark Public Library, the New Jersey Historical Society Library, the New Jersey State Library, the New Jersey Academy of Medicine Library, the Rutgers University Library, the New York University Library, the New York Academy of Medicine Library, the New York Public Library, and the National Library of Medicine. I am especially indebted to the following staff members of the Newark Public Library New Jersey Reference Division, for their tireless support: Gertrude Cahalan, Senior Librarian; Robert Blackwell, Senior Librarian; and Charles F. Cummings, Principal Librarian. Financial assistance was provided during the initial period of my research by the Josiah Macy, Jr., Foundation through its fellowship program in the History of Medicine and Biological Sciences. An excellent job of typing the manuscript was done by Mrs. Shirley Williams.

Chapter 5, "Passaic Valley Trunk Sewer," was previously published in *New Jersey History* (Winter 1970) and is reproduced by permission of The New Jersey Historical Society.

In researching and writing the book I have benefited from the advice of many colleagues and friends. Professors Bayrd Still and Brooke Hindle first interested me in the subject of urban public health while I was a graduate student at New York University. Professor James Harvey Young of Emory University read the manuscript in its entirety and made many valuable suggestions. Any faults in content and style are, needless to say, my own.

NOTES

1. John B. Blake, *Public Health in the Town of Boston: 1630-1822* (Cambridge: Harvard University Press, 1959), p. vii.
2. See Dorothy T. Scanlon, "The Public Health Movement in Boston, 1870-1910" (Unpublished Ph.D. diss., Boston University, 1956).

Safeguarding
the
Public Health

1

The Nation's Unhealthiest City

The nation's unhealthiest city. That was the judgment made on Newark by the United States Census of 1890. Newark's death rate was 27.4 per 1,000 persons, highest in the nation of any city of over 100,000 population. The 28 largest American cities had a cumulative death rate of only 21.6 per 1,000 persons. Hence Newark, whose population was 182,000, had incurred over 1,000 excessive deaths.[1] Newark led the nation in deaths from scarlet fever, in infant mortality, and in deaths of children under five years of age. It ranked among the top ten in typhoid fever, malaria, tuberculosis, and diphtheria and croup (laryngitis).

Newark's mortality experience ran counter to the trend of urban death rates in the late nineteenth century. In the years 1860-1880 death rates in American cities generally fell from approximately 25 to 40 per 1,000 population to about 15 to 25. Of the large urban centers, only four Southern cities and Newark continued to have mortality rates of over 30 per 1,000 population.[2] Moreover, Newark's death rate was higher than it had been before the Civil War.[3]

Paradoxically, Newark's decline in public health occurred during a period of prosperity. Newark emerged from the Civil War a major industrial center. More than half of Newark's wage earners in 1880 were employed in industry. Several new industries achieved prominence, including chemicals, electrical machinery, and smelting and refining, revealing a shift from workshop to factory and from individually crafted wares to mass produced goods. Financial institutions followed industry, helping to balance the economy.[4] In the words of Newark's official biographer, it was "An Age of Giants," an age of daring entrepreneurs who established great businesses, and of inventors like Edward Wetson, inventor of the "Normal Cell," and John Wesley Hyatt, inventor of celluloid, whose discoveries changed the lives of all Americans.[5]

Foreign-born immigrants provided the muscle for Newark's factories.

3

Nearness to New York City, the nation's largest port of entry, and the opportunities afforded unskilled labor in industry and municipal construction attracted large numbers of immigrants to Newark. The percentage of foreign-born in Newark in the years 1870-1910 fluctuated between 29 and 34 percent. Along with their American-born children, the foreign element made up nearly half of the city's population.[6]

The Irish, who were first brought to Newark in the 1820s to build the Morris Canal, lived principally in the low-lying "Down Neck" area bordering the Passaic River and the Newark salt meadows. This malaria-infested area became the traditional center of Newark's immigrant population. In the late 1840s and 1850s the Irish were joined by German immigrants. Skill, thrift, and hard work soon won for the Germans an important place in the city's economy. The largest immigrant group, they also became a potent force in municipal politics. After the Civil War, successful Germans began moving to the "Hill," the country heights lying to the west and northwest of downtown Newark. Here they established a distinctively German community complete with beer gardens, gymnasiums, and singing societies. About 1890 Italians, Slavs, Russian Jews, and other immigrant groups from southern and eastern Europe began supplanting the older ethnic stocks from northern and western Europe.[7]

Like the groups that had preceded them, the new immigrants settled in "Down Neck," or "Ironbound," as it was now called (because of the iron foundries and the Pennsylvania Railroad tracks that girded the area). "Ironbound" also attracted industrialists eager to take advantage of the region's superb rail and water facilities. Soon the combination of heavy industry and tenements made "Ironbound" Newark's worst slum. The inner wards situated between "Ironbound" and the "Hill" contained the best residential areas. Fine homes were built in downtown Newark, commanding views overlooking Washington and Military parks. Other wealthy residents made their homes on South Broad Street and on the ends of the ridge running along High Street.

Streetcars radically altered the city's residential patterns. The appearance of first the horse-drawn and later the electric trolley prompted an exodus of affluent workers from the inner wards. The cheap land opened up for settlement by the trolley made it possible for commuters to work at good jobs in the city while living in the country. With the arrival of the first wave of southern and eastern European immigrants in the 1890s, the movement to the suburbs accelerated. Fearful of being submerged in an alien sea, native Americans deserted the city in droves. Residential sections that lost their middle-class inhabitants either were rezoned for business or were taken over by the newcomers.[8]

Not all native residents fled the arrival of the new immigrants: some could not afford a house in the suburbs, and some had business interests that kept them downtown with the newcomers. The old, the sick, the unsuccessful, and others trapped in the city were forced to live in tenements and lodging houses. Young families stayed in the city until they had accumulated enough money to put a down payment on a suburban house. Wealthy industrialists desirous of being near their businesses, and able to isolate themselves from the discomforts and pathologies of city life, also stayed behind. The view of downtown Newark presented a discordant juxtaposition of fine homes and ugly tenements and factories, though increasingly work and residence were becoming separated.[9]

Newark in this period began to take on the look and characteristics of a bustling industrial center. Overhead, telephone and power lines crisscrossed, hiding the city in a cobweb of wires, while below, trolleys speeded commuters to and from the suburbs. Department stores were opened, and two outstanding newspapers, the *Sunday Call* and the *Newark Evening News,* were begun. Casting aside the conservative tradition of the Newark press, the new journals offered sprightly, independent news reporting attuned to the variety of tastes of urban readers. By 1900 the *Sunday Call* was publishing editions of sixty pages with feature articles, theater columns, and sport and fashion pages, and was acknowledged to be one of New Jersey's most influential newspapers. Similarly, the *News,* by relying less on lengthy and frequently dated foreign dispatches and more on investigative journalism of local events, swamped its more staid competitors and quickly became Newark's largest circulating daily.[10]

Yet amidst all these signs of progress, life in Newark had soured. Sickness and premature death were depriving Newarkers of the fruits of their labors. Growth, urbanization, and industrialization had been recklessly pushed forward without a corresponding expansion of health and welfare services, and the city was now having to pay the cost. A newspaper editor in 1857 summed up the city's lopsided development by noting that there were forty churches but not one hospital; by then Newark's population was approaching 60,000. A dispensary was established the following year in the offices of the city's newly organized board of health. At the dispensary drugs were furnished and the poor were vaccinated against smallpox. Persons too sick to travel were treated in their homes by district physicians attached to the dispensary. Though these instruments of community medicine served a large clientele, they did not take the place of a hospital.[11]

The absence of a hospital in Newark resulted in many hardships for its citizens, especially the laboring classes. Most importantly, there was no medical center equipped to handle the daily accidents that occurred in the city's railroad yards and workshops. Consequently, workers injured on the job had to be rushed from one doctor's office to another in a frantic search for emergency treatment. Sick persons who could no longer support themselves were shipped to the almshouse, where they were indiscriminately bedded down with drunkards, criminals, and the feeble-minded, often two or more to a bed. Because of the absence of a hospital, individuals recovering from serious illnesses seldom were able to obtain proper nursing care. Finally, citizens needing surgery or specialized medical treatment were compelled to go to New York City to find it.[12]

For nearly two hundred years following its founding in 1666, Newark sponged off the medical resources of its neighbor across the Hudson River. In the late 1850s an abortive attempt was made to establish a municipal hospital. The failure of the plan prompted the city health officer to remark that the want of a hospital "has been a reproach to our people, an injustice to those who might properly demand attention at our hands, and a burden to the charities of our neighbors."[13]

The holocaust of the Civil War led to the founding of Newark's first hospital. Medical care centers were desperately needed for returning injured soldiers. When trains began bringing back the first wounded to Newark on May 10, 1862, Marcus L. Ward, the Republican political leader of New Jersey (popularly known as the "Soldiers' Friend" for his efforts in obtaining pensions and other relief for wounded soldiers and the families of killed soldiers), assumed the responsibility for organizing a hospital. With money borrowed from the New Jersey state government, Ward leased a four-story brick warehouse on Centre Street, between the New Jersey Railroad and the Passaic River. In just two days the building was scrubbed, fumigated, outfitted with hospital equipment and readied for occupancy. At its peak of operation the hospital contained 17 pavilions housing 1,020 beds. The hospital was closed in the summer of 1865 and the facility converted into a state soldiers' home.[14]

The advantages of a hospital, however, were not lost on the people of

Newark, and within five years of the closing of Ward Hospital, three private hospitals were established. St. Barnabas, an institution affiliated with the Episcopal Church, was opened in 1864 but was not incorporated until 1867. In 1869 The Sisters of the Poor of St. Francis, a German order, founded St. Michael's Hospital. Clara Maass Hospital ("German Hospital") was started in 1870 by German fraternal and benevolent organizations. Though church affiliated, the hospitals served persons of all races, creeds, and ethnic groups. A few specialized facilities were also established, such as the Home for Incurables and Convalescents, a private forty-eight bed home for women, and the Newark Eye and Ear Infirmary, which was partly supported with municipal funds.[15]

The city paid each hospital $2,500 annually for the use of ten beds. Public aid to church affiliated institutions was contrary to the American tradition of the separation of church and state, leading the *Newark Daily Advertiser* to seek the establishment of a municipal hospital. Finally, in 1882 Newark City Hospital was opened. The first annual report of the Board of Directors stated that the hospital was to be "devoted exclusively to the treatment and relief of the indigent sick and disabled." The charity stigma attached to the institution was further apparent in its location in a wing of the almshouse.[16]

Lack of adequate facilities for treating the sick poor was only one indicator of the city's business priorities. The material progress of Newark during the late nineteenth century had been purchased at the cost of a ravaged environment and an increase in morbidity and mortality. Alarm over the city's worsening sanitary condition led one Newark newspaper to declare:

> Our weekly mortality reports show the outbreaks from time to time of preventable diseases in certain quarters, easily traceable to direct violations of the rules of health, and the ratio of death is generally above the average of our sister cities. If further evidence was needed we have only to use our eyes and noses to discover abounding causes.[17]

An earlier concern for the hazards of crowded community life was sacrificed in the heedless pursuit of profits and growth. The water supply was drawn from the polluted Passaic River, and sewers emptied into sluggish tidal creeks not far from major centers of population. The smell of excreta decomposing in the sun, and of the Passaic River when the water level was low, forced residents to keep their windows closed on even the most muggy summer nights. From spring through fall hordes of mosquitoes took flight from the meadows, making life in the city at night unbearable. The death rate hovered at about 25 per 1,000 population and at no time before 1895 was less than 20 per 1,000 population.[18] Three times during the 1870s the mortality rate reached 30 per 1,000 population as a result of epidemics of smallpox and diphtheria.

But if epidemic diseases were responsible for the high peaks in the death rate curve, endemic diseases caused the most fatalities. Tuberculosis, diseases of infancy, and respiratory and intestinal diseases were the major causes of death.[19] Surprisingly, these diseases generated little excitement. Because they were commonplace, they were not as feared as smallpox and diphtheria. Familiarity led to a casual acceptance of these undercurrents of death.

Tuberculosis was preeminently the disease of the Industrial Revolution. In the dingy sweatshops, the dusty factories, the sunless and ill-ventilated tenements, and wherever else the working poor were found, the disease flourished. Few among the poor had the physical strength to withstand an attack of the white plague. The physical and spiritual exhaustion brought on by malnutrition and oppressive living conditions rendered the poor an easy prey. In 1881 tuberculosis accounted for about 16 percent of Newark's fatalities.[20]

The association of tenement housing with tuberculosis was borne out by the census of 1890. The three wards in Newark having death rates from tuberculosis of over 400 per 100,000 population were described as follows: "a manufacturing section, with residents in very moderate circumstances"; "principally cheap tenements occupied, for the great part, by Irish"; "principally tenements of a poor class." By way of contrast the eighth ward, which had the lowest death rate, 229.89 per 100,000 population, was said to contain "a mixed population of the middle class plus the finest residential section of the city."[21]

Water supply was a problem which affected equally all segments of society. In need of a vastly enlarged water supply, Newark turned to the Passaic River at just the same time (1870) that neighboring communities and factories started using the waterway as a repository for their wastes. A contaminated water supply coupled with faulty sewerage led to an increase in the incidence of water-borne diseases. Gastrointestinal ailments beset citizens, and the typhoid fever mortality rate arched steadily upward until it attained a height municipal leaders could not ignore with impunity.[22]

The innocent suffered most from Newark's negligence. Diseases of
infancy were the city's leading cause of death. Infant deaths in 1881
accounted for 21 percent of all Newark fatalities. Almost two out of every
ten infants died before their first birthday.[23] The reasons for this frightful
slaughter were apparent. The water used to wash the infant's bottle was
polluted, while the milk on which he was weaned came from diseased
and emaciated cows and was produced on dairies which in their sanitary
maintenance resembled pigsties.

Judging from the mortality and morbidity statistics, children must have
been continually sick. Measles, chickenpox, mumps, rubella, whooping
cough, scarlet fever, and diphtheria were rampant, and it was a rare mother
who could not recount the upbringing of her child by recalling the ages
at which little Johnny had come down with red spots, pustules, or
swollen glands. Scarlet fever and diphtheria, because of their frightful
symptoms and high mortality, caused the greatest anxiety and grief. Acute
infectious diseases of childhood together with malaria, typhoid fever,
and smallpox were responsible in 1881 (a nonepidemic year) for one-
seventh of all fatalities. Respiratory illnesses affected all ages and accounted for about 12 percent of Newark's mortality. Other important
causes of death included brain and spinal diseases and diseases of the
heart and circulatory systems.[24]

Parsimony and partisanship at one time or another imperiled every
city service. "Police and fire departments were dangerously undermanned
and subjected to such petty political control that they verged often on
the edge of breakdown."[25] The common council, which until 1891
retained control of most administrative services, lacked the expertise
demanded by the increasing complexity of urban government. Though
Newark was relatively free of graft and corruption, at least when compared to its neighbors, city services failed to keep pace with municipal
growth. There were simply too many improvements to be made at a
time when the paramount concern of the city fathers was to keep taxes
low so as to attract new business. What services were provided were
unplanned.[26]

Newark's patchwork administrative services and niggardly attitude
toward public improvements caused it to become one of the nation's
most unsanitary cities. Only 49 miles of sewers existed in Newark in
1883 as contrasted with 131 miles of improved streets. About two-thirds
of the city's residents, including a great number of those living in the

central downtown area, were dependent upon privies and cesspools. A sanitary investigation made that year disclosed the widespread existence of broken drains, garbage-strewn streets, and gutters made repulsive by decomposed kitchen slops and washwater.[27]

The filth that befouled Newark was not only unsightly, but dangerous. Many of the privies were made of wood or had open bottoms and sides, permitting their contents to contaminate the surrounding soil. As a result, people who drank from wells were plagued with dysentery and typhoid fever. Newark's poor sanitary state is particularly revealing of the low regard in which life was held by municipal leaders, since it was believed then that decomposing filth was responsible for high mortality rates.[28]

For over two decades following its creation in 1857, the Newark Board of Health, which had the responsibility of overseeing sanitary conditions, lay moribund. The average annual expenditure of the board during the years 1870-1880 was $9,000, or barely $.07 per capita. A corporal's guard of one meat inspector and four sanitary inspectors comprised the field force of the department. Inspections were made only upon complaint; the board made no independent investigations of its own. Even when nuisances were uncovered, prosecution of malefactors was haphazard.[29] The secretary of the American Public Health Association in 1875 reported that Newark's sanitary government was "a fiction."[30]

Politics partly accounted for the board of health's ineffectiveness. Political retainers were put to work as nuisance abators and street cleaners. Men without the intelligence or agility to be schoolteachers, policemen, or firemen were given jobs pushing brooms and loading carts. Appointment to the department was made on the basis of whom, rather than what, one knew. Every change in political administration witnessed a large turnover in personnel.[31] Consequently, the department was saddled with a succession of incompetent inspectors. In 1883 Newark's health officer was quoted as saying that the men employed in his department were "totally unfit to perform the duties . . . assigned to them."[32]

Newark lacked the imagination and boldness displayed by other cities in meeting urban problems. The temper of the community was too conservative for its own welfare. Aside from business matters, petty issues dominated the public forum. Thus when German residents attempted to visit beer gardens and stage festivals on the Sabbath, they incurred the wrath of Protestant ministers. A bitter controversy ensued, and for a number of years the issue was the focal point of the city's mayoralty elections.[33] While Newarkers wrestled with their consciences, they lived in filth; blue laws, prohibition, and other such moral dilemmas weighed more on their minds than the thousand persons who yearly perished of preventable diseases.

NOTES

1. 27.4-21.6 x 182,000/1,000. U.S. Bureau of the Census, *Eleventh Census of the United States, 1890: Report on Vital and Social Statistics*, II, 2-4, 21-22, 75, 78, 85, 88, 96, 99.

2. The high mortality rates of Southern cities is attributable to epidemics of yellow fever, malaria, the presence of large numbers of blacks, whose death rate considerably exceeded that of whites, and the general backwardness of the South during this period. Newark's high mortality rate is less easy to explain. Partly it may be accounted for by the city's rapid growth after the Civil War. But other cities were also undergoing industrialization and had large immigrant populations. Some of Newark's health problems, such as malaria and a contaminated water supply, were rooted in the geography of the Newark area. Then too, the reporting of vital statistics at this time was not a scientific process, and communities reluctant to admit to excessive deaths could easily distort their actual mortality experience.

3. Howard D. Kramer, "History of the Public Health Movement in the United States, 1850 to 1900" (Unpublished Ph.D. diss., State University of Iowa, 1942), pp. 182-3.

4. Samuel Harry Popper, "Newark, N.J., 1870-1910: Chapters in the Evolution of an American Metropolis" (Unpublished Ph.D. diss., New York University, 1952), pp. 13-14.

5. John T. Cunningham, *Newark* (Newark: The New Jersey Historical Society, 1966), pp. 174-84.

6. Ibid., pp. 201-8; Popper, "Newark," pp. 63, 126-35.

7. Popper, "Newark," pp. 160-5.

8. Ibid., pp. 166-71.

9. Ibid., pp. 173-5; Newark, Board of Education, *Newark Study Leaflets* (1914), No. 37, *Newark Advantages*, p. 2.

10. Cunningham, *Newark*, pp. 189-96; Popper, "Newark," pp. 223-28.

11. *Newark Daily Advertiser*, March 17, June 5, 1857; *Charter of Newark and Revised Ordinances* (1858), *1857 Charter of the City of Newark*, pp. 23, 167-73.

12. *Newark Daily Advertiser*, October 27, 1853, December 30, 1854, March 17, April 30, June 5, December 14, 1857, February 14, 1859, as cited in Samuel Berg (comp.), "Medical Practice and Hospital Development in Newark, N.J., 1850-1887, as Reported in Newark Daily Advertiser," Newark Public Library, New Jersey Reference Division.

13. Newark, *Reports of the Health Physician, Secretary of the Dispensary Board, and the District Physicians to the Board of Health, together with the Plan of Organization of the Newark City Dispensary, 1860* (Newark: Newark Daily Advertiser, 1860), p. 34.

14. David L. Pierson, *Narratives of Newark, 1866-1916* (Newark: Pierson Publishing Co., 1917), pp. 299-302.

15. Rosary S. Gilheany, "Early Newark Hospitals," *Proceedings of the New Jersey Historical Society* (January 1965), pp. 10-24; Frank John Urquhart, *A History of the City of Newark, New Jersey* (3 vols.; New York: The Lewis Historical Publishing Co., 1913), II, 63.

16. Urquhart, *Newark*, I, 63; *Newark Daily Advertiser*, August 12, 1882, November 21, 1884, as cited in Berg, "Medical Practice in Newark"; David L. Cowen, *Medicine and Health in New Jersey: A History*, Vol. XVI of *The New Jersey Historical Series*, eds. Richard M. Huber and Wheaton J. Lane (Princeton, N.J.: D. Van Nostrand Co., Inc., 1964), pp. 96, 98; Newark, *The Mayor's Message, Together with the Reports of the City Officers of the City of Newark, N.J., 1881, Board of Health*, p. 408, *1883, Newark City Hospital*, p. 672. Some reports of city officers were published separately as well. When a report of a city department that was published together with the mayor's message is quoted, the citation will appear as follows: *Newark Annual Reports, year, name of reporting unit.*

17. *Newark Daily Advertiser*, June 14, 1883.

18. Below, Appendix.

19. Ibid.

20. Ezra M. Hunt, "A Study of Consumption as a Preventable Disease," New Jersey Board of Health, *Annual Report for 1881*, p. 245 (hereinafter referred to as *ARNJBH*).

21. U.S. Bureau of the Census, *Eleventh Census of the United States, 1890: Report on Vital and Social Statistics*, I, 588, II, 276-83.

22. Ezra Mundy Hunt, "The Passaic River as Related to Water Supply and Death Rates," *ARNJBH, 1887*, pp. 317-58.

23. Below, Appendix.

24. Ibid.

25. Cunningham, *Newark*, p. 222.

26. Ibid., pp. 222-3; Popper, "Newark," p. 270.

27. *Newark Daily Advertiser*, August 7, 9, 11, 1883.

28. Ibid., September 1, 1883.

29. U.S. Bureau of the Census, *Tenth Census of the United States, 1880: Social Statistics of Cities,* Pt. I, pp. 711-2; *Newark Annual Reports, 1879, Board of Health,* pp. 403-8, *1880,* pp. 427-41.

30. Elisha Harris, "Report on the Public Health Service in the Principal Cities, and the Progress of the Sanitary Works in the United States," American Public Health Association, *Public Health Reports and Papers,* II (1874-1875), 169.

31. *Newark Evening News,* March 13, 1884.

32. Ibid., November 6, 1883.

33. Popper, "Newark," pp. 79-85.

2

A City Comes of Age

If the era 1865-1895 was an age of entrepreneurial capitalism in which the pursuit of wealth took precedence over all other concerns, then the years 1895-1918 were a time of nascent maturity during which the city began to assume greater responsibility for safeguarding the public health. During these years, Newark changed from an industrial city to a metropolis. Swelled by a flood of immigrants from southern and eastern Europe, Newark's population mushroomed from 182,000 in 1890 to 430,000 in 1918. The city grew outwardly as well, incorporating neighboring Clinton Township and Vailsburg. With still further annexations contemplated, city leaders envisioned the emergence of a greater Newark metropolitan area embracing all of northern New Jersey between the Passaic River and the Orange Mountains.[1]

In Newark and throughout the nation, the reins of the economy passed from industrial magnates to impersonal financial institutions. Newark benefited from the triumph of finance capitalism, for it was the home of two of the nation's best-known life insurance companies: Prudential Insurance Company and Mutual Benefit Life Insurance Company. By 1895 Newark was surpassed only by Hartford, Philadelphia, and New York City in insurance assets. In addition, several of New Jersey's best-known corporations, including the Public Service Corporation and New Jersey Bell Telephone Company, made Newark their corporate headquarters. Though it still boasted of its diversified manufacturing, Newark was becoming a white collar community.[2]

Change was manifest in the appearance of the skyline. Steeples became dwarfed by skyscrapers which sprang up in the downtown business area. Concrete, glass, and steel were substituted for wood, brick, and iron. Gargoyles, domed windows, and other architectural ornaments gradually began to give way to the sparse rectangular symmetry that has become so dominant a feature of urban landscapes. Fortunately, the city preserved

a few distinguished church edifices from an earlier age. The city also
erected a number of gracious public buildings with marble pillars,
elegant staircases, and rotundas. The clutter of the industrial city was
removed. Wires went underground and dangerous grade crossings were
eliminated, thereby improving public safety while beautifying the city.
Electric light replaced gas light, and asphalt was substituted for brick,
granite blocks, and cobblestones—just in time for the coming of the
automobile.[3]

Three- and four-story tenement houses appeared in Newark about
1890. Into these dark, airless apartments were crowded immigrant
families and their relatives and friends.[4] But the closely knit ethnic
communities in which the immigrants lived had redeeming virtues,
for they provided a safe base from which immigrants could find their
way into the mainstream of American life. For many immigrants a
tenement district was only a way station on the road to a better life, if
not for themselves, then for their children.

Newark started to acquire the social, intellectual, and cultural ac-
coutrements befitting a metropolitan center. A public library system
evolved, and a city museum was opened. Under the direction of John
Cotton Dana, "probably the most famous public librarian this country
has known,"[5] the library became an integral part of the community.
Foreign language literature was introduced into the branch libraries,
where immigrants were encouraged to read in both their native language
and English. So popular was the idea that often there were lines to enter
the libraries. The institutional church and the settlement house also
began their careers in Newark about this time.[6]

The years 1895-1918 were a time of reform in American life, usually
referred to as the Progressive Era. In Newark, Progressivism manifested
itself principally in the quest for a modern and efficient government.
To this end per capita spending was increased, the mayor's powers were
enhanced, and municipal functions were extended into new areas. In
1911 a City Plan Commission was appointed to project Newark's future
development. The desire for accountability and expertness in municipal
administration prompted a vigorous home rule movement and led in 1917
to the creation of a commission form of government.[7]

Nowhere was the city's coming of age better reflected than in the vital
statistics compiled annually by the city clerk and by the board of health.
The period 1895-1922 witnessed Newark's greatest advance in public
health. Newark's death rate in 1922 was 12.1 per 1,000 population, nearly

60 percent less than it was in 1890.[8] Among the factors responsible for the change were: important medical discoveries, especially the germ theory of disease, technological innovations, improved living conditions, and decisive government action to protect the public health.

The years 1895-1900 form a watershed in the history of the Newark Board of Health. After a decade of floundering, the board began to right itself and to take its proper place alongside other agencies of city government. By 1900 the board had gained public acceptance and had won the respect of the people of Newark.

Boards of health throughout the nation were revitalized in the 1890s by the advent of bacteriology. Through use of pasteurization, treatment of water and sewerage, and vaccines and serums, several of mankind's most fearful scourges were virtually eradicated. Besides enhancing the prestige of public health work, the germ theory of disease also forced the young discipline to become more professional. The realization that sense perceptions were unreliable in detecting microscopic dangers placed a premium on scientific procedures. As public health became the province of the sanitary engineer, the chemist, and the bacteriologist, departments of public health were exempted from political interference.[9]

Able leadership, an intangible but vital factor in the board's resurrection, came in 1892 with the appointment of Herman Christopher Henry Herold as president and David D. Chandler as health officer. For the next twenty years Chandler and Herold guided the destiny of the Newark Board of Health. Together they cajoled and educated politicians and the public alike about needed reforms and increased powers and expenditures.[10] The board of health was also attracting trained professionals to fill key positions within the department, many of whom made the department their life's work. More than thirty years of service each were rendered by Herbert B. Baldwin, the chemist, Dr. Richard N. Connolly, the chief bacteriologist, and Dr. Edward E. Worl, the superintendent of the bureau of contagious diseases and first medical director of the Newark sanatorium at Verona.

Under the direction of Chandler and Herold, the Newark Board of Health made a fresh start. The sanitary reforms proposed by the board in the late nineteenth century were quietly completed. Privies were banned, polluted wells were closed, and sewerage was extended throughout the city except for the meadows. Devoid of human presence, the meadows were not in need of a sewage disposal system until World War I, when

war plants were established there; and then, because of the watery sub-
soil, septic tanks had to be used.[11] In 1895 a bacteriological laboratory
was established, and in 1904 mosquito extermination work was begun.
Most gratifying of all to the members of the board, the mortality rate
plummeted from the ignominious pinnacle of 1890. Commenting on "the
great decrease in the [Newark] death rate," the 1900 census reported it
was "attributed generally to the advanced policies of the board of health
along the lines of preventive medicine."[12]

Some of the remedies to Newark's sanitary problems were shortsighted.
When Newark in 1889 turned to the Pequannock River for its drinking
water, the city lost its incentive for cleansing the Passaic River. Newark
along with other communities in the lower Passaic River Valley continued
to discharge raw sewage into the waterway, creating an intolerable nuisance.
Similarly, Newark and the cities of northeastern New Jersey solved their
waste disposal problem by dumping their garbage on the Hackensack and
Newark meadows.

Problems of environmental sanitation transcend the interests and
capabilities of cities, necessitating a regional approach. Recognizing the
limitations of local governments, New Jersey early in the twentieth century
established district and state sewerage and water supply commissions.
Reclamation of the Hackensack meadows, however, was held up by quarreling among the concerned communities.[13]

The board of health was eminently successful in ridding the city of
disease-bearing insects. The mosquito, which had been the bane of
Newark residents for nearly two and one-half centuries, was finally brought
under control.[14] Similarly, a successful attack was made against the
household fly, a filthy pest and transmitter of intestinal diseases. The
city's fecal deposits and organic wastes were a magnet for flies. The
thoroughfares bordering Military Park, one of Newark's most densely
populated sections, received the excrement of a thousand horses and other
animals daily. Moreover, stables could frequently be found behind
tenements.[15]

Following the discovery by New York City health officials in 1914
that flies contributed to the incidence of summer diarrhea in infants, a
vigorous fly extermination campaign was begun. Livestock owners were
required to fit manure basins with fly-tight covers and to cement and
drain stable floors. Property owners were compelled to keep rented
premises screened and garbage cans closed. But the efforts of the Newark

Board of Health to eliminate the breeding areas of the household fly
would probably have come to naught had not technology come to the
board's aid. With the replacement of animals by machines and the substitution of chemical fertilizer for manure, the unsightly manure pile along
with the flies it attracted, both on the farm and in the city, became a
thing of the past.[16]

Notable strides were made in enhancing the wholesomeness of the
food supply. Here again technological advances were of immeasurable
benefit to urban dwellers. The growing use of canning and refrigeration
prevented spoilage, made for a more varied diet, and insured the availability of nutritious foods the year around. The Newark Board of Health
intensified its efforts to insure the safety and quality of foodstuffs,
though its work in this area still left much to be desired. The milk supply
was scrutinized and greatly improved.[17] Slaughterhouses, markets, and
restaurants were regularly inspected and scored on their sanitary condition. And in 1917 an ordinance was introduced requiring food handlers
to undergo examination for communicable diseases.[18]

The most significant public health development of the period was the
conquest of acute, communicable diseases which, with the exceptions of
tuberculosis and pneumonia, ceased to be a major factor in the death rate.
Better methods of vaccination brought smallpox under control, while
the discovery of diphtheria antitoxin did the same for that disease.
Scarlet fever, on the other hand, was rendered innocuous without any
noteworthy assist from man. A minor ailment in the colonial and early
national periods, the disease suddenly became virulent about 1840, and
for the next sixty years rivaled diphtheria in destructiveness. Then, for
unknown reasons, it began to decline in potency, becoming once again a
mild childhood sickness (in most instances).[19]

With the introduction of Pequannock water, the threat of typhoid
fever receded, but because of infection occurring outside the city, the
disease could not be totally eradicated. Nearly all of the cases occurred
in late summer and early fall among returning summer vacationers who,
while in the countryside, had drunk from polluted wells or had consumed
food fertilized with night soil. The disease was also kept alive by carriers,
especially unclean food handlers who worked in private homes and
restaurants. In 1917 smallpox, typhoid fever, and infectious diseases of
childhood accounted for only 2.35 percent of Newark's mortality, down
83 percent from 1881.[20]

Facilities for the sick poor continued to develop along the lines established in the decades following the Civil War. As new ethnic groups gained
in number and wealth, they established their own medical charities. There
was, however, an important change in the nature of hospitals. The development of safe surgical techniques coupled with the growing ability of
physicians to cure illness transformed hospitals from nursing institutions
into places of healing. When the effectiveness of hospitals became apparent,
their numbers greatly increased. Among the hospitals opened in Newark
during this period were: Beth Israel Hospital (incorporated 1901), St.
James Hospital (incorporated 1891), The Presbyterian Hospital in Newark,
New Jersey (incorporated 1909), and The Homeopathic Hospital of
Essex County (incorporated 1903). Special hospitals and medical facilities
were also started for babies, crippled children, expectant mothers, and
incurables. To permit patients to go to hospitals of their own religious
faith, the city maintained the practice of renting beds in private institutions;
besides, the annual rental fee of $250 per bed was a bargain.[21]

Though intended as medical charities, a number of beds were set aside
in church-affiliated hospitals for paying patients who were admitted
through their family physicians. As the cost of hospital equipment skyrocketed, voluntary hospitals became increasingly dependent upon the
fees of nonindigent patients. This in turn forced the hospitals to go beyond
their minimal obligation to treat sickness. To keep their paying patients
happy, voluntary hospitals had to start offering middle-class amenities
and personalized medical care.[22]

The municipal hospital, Newark's main health care facility, in 1918
had four hundred beds, all free, plus an emergency out-patient department
for treatment of minor injuries. Admission to the hospital was by permit
of a City Physician, by application to the Newark Board of Health or the
overseer of the poor, or by direct application to the hospital. Though the
hospital provided excellent treatment, mostly of a major medical nature,
it manifested the defects inherent in philanthropic medicine. Newark
City Hospital was poorly financed and was run according to the priorities
set by the administrators and by the medical staff. Humanitarianism and
the Hippocratic Oath assured the poor, in most instances, of the latest
treatments medical science had to offer. That, however, was as far as the
hospital's excellence extended. Unlike voluntary hospitals, medical charities
were under no compulsion to take into account the human needs and
comforts of their patients. Because health care was not viewed as one of

an American's rights, public opinion opposed providing for the poor the same comprehensive medical care available to those able to pay their own way. Thus, despite the rental by the city of 123 beds in private institutions, Newark City Hospital was packed to the rafters. Patients with medical and nervous disorders were confined to poorly lighted and unventilated basement wards where they were denied the opportunity of exercise and recreation. The patients' clothing, hung on racks in basement rooms, frequently was torn or soiled. Though the hospital had been specifically established to provide relief for the indigent sick and disabled, to make room for new patients, convalescents who had no one to nurse them were sent to the almshouse.[23]

The city dispensary, comprising clinics in general medicine, the medical specialties, and programs adopted by the board of health (for tuberculosis, child hygiene, venereal disease), gave medical advice and supplied medicines free or for a small fee. Though clinical medicine experienced great growth in the years 1880-1920, it was poor man's medicine, hedged about with restrictions designed to place it out of competition with private practice.[24] Thus a person with dental caries could not have his cavities filled at the city dispensary; and rather than pay for expensive private dental care, he frequently ignored them. Similarly, illnesses detected at the board of health's Baby Keep-Well stations had to be treated privately. It is likely that the quality of clinic medicine declined as medical training and research became centered in hospitals. Young physicians who once sought clinical experience in dispensaries now opted for the more prestigious hospital internships or else used their clinic service as a steppingstone to a hospital appointment. Also, the clinics were located in the Newark Public Health Department building, when logically they should have been a part of the city hospital's out-patient department.[25]

Three dental clinics operating under the supervision of a private dental clinic association furnished free treatment for children sixteen or under. The clinics, which were organized under state law, received an annual appropriation from the city of $10,000, and were used mainly by children referred to them from the public schools. Rounding out the medical care provided the sick poor in Newark, there were six part-time City Physicians who treated persons confined to their homes. The physicians also were supposed to report on sanitary conditions in their districts. A vestigial remnant of nineteenth-century community medicine, the work of the

City Physicians was poorly supervised and was not coordinated with other health care services.[26]

Newark during the years 1895-1918 began to use the wealth generated by industrialization to provide its citizens with an expanded array of social-welfare services. Libraries were opened, and a county park system was established. The city was rid of revolting filth which in the past had provided a nursery for disease. Several acute communicable diseases were all but vanquished and hospital facilities were expanded. In the forefront of the forces striving to make the city a safer and better place in which to live was the Newark Board of Health.

NOTES

1. Samuel Harry Popper, "Newark, N.J., 1870-1910: Chapters in the Evolution of an American Metropolis" (Unpublished Ph.D. diss., New York University, 1952), pp. 442-3.

2. John T. Cunningham, *Newark* (Newark: The New Jersey Historical Society, 1966), pp. 185-8; Popper, "Newark," pp. 89-96.

3. Cunningham, *Newark*, pp. 227-8, 232-40.

4. Popper, "Newark," pp. 175-8.

5. Cunningham, *Newark*, p. 220.

6. Ibid., pp. 220, 240; Popper, "Newark," pp. 217, 415-25.

7. Popper, "Newark," pp. 269-71, 435-41; J. Wilmer Kennedy, *Newark in the Public Schools of Newark: A Course of Study on Newark, its Geography, Civics and History, with Biographical Sketches and a Reference Index* (Newark: Newark Board of Education, 1911), pp. 59-60; Cunningham, *Newark*, p. 262,

8. Below, Appendix.

9. Barbara Gutman Rosenkrantz, *Public Health and the State: Changing Views in Massachusetts, 1842-1936* (Cambridge: Harvard University Press, 1972), p. 126.

10. *Sunday Call*, June 8, 1913.

11. *Newark Annual Reports, 1915, Board of Health*, p. 985, *1916*, pp. 1, 273.

12. U.S. Bureau of the Census, *Twelfth Census of the United States, 1900, Vital Statistics*, III, Pt. I, 59, 62.

13. Below, Chapters 4 and 5.

14. Below, Chapter 6.

15. Milton J. Rosenau, *Preventive Medicine and Hygiene* (1st ed.; New York: D. Appleton and Co., 1913), pp. 91-2; *Newark Annual Reports,*

1871, Mayor's Message, p. 20; George B. Ford and E. P. Goodrich, *Housing Report,* [Reports of] *The City Plan Commission, Newark, N.J.* (Newark: Mathias Plum, 1913), pp. 9, 14-15.

16. *Newark Annual Reports, 1915, Board of Health,* pp. 979-80, *1918,* p. 209; Wilson G. Smillie, *Public Health, Its Promise for the Future: A Chronicle of the Development of Public Health in the United States, 1607-1914* (New York: The Macmillan Co., 1955), pp. 353-4.

17. Below, Chapter VII.

18. Samuel C. Prescott, "Food Conservation," *A Half Century of Public Health: Jubilee Historical Volume of the American Public Health Association,* ed. Mazÿck Porcher Ravenel (New York: American Public Health Association, 1921), pp. 221-35; *Newark Daily Advertiser,* April 14, May 2, 1885; *Newark Evening News,* May 28, 1917.

19. John Duffy, *Epidemics in Colonial America* (Baton Rouge, La.: Louisiana State University Press, 1953), p. 137; Rosenau, *Preventive Medicine,* 8th ed., pp. 73-74; *Newark Annual Reports, 1916 Board of Health,* pp. 1, 230-1.

20. Below, Appendix.

21. A. W. MacDougall, *The Philanthropies of Newark, New Jersey: A Descriptive Directory* (n.p., 1916), pp. 22-29; Bureau of Municipal Research, New York, "A Survey of the Government, Finances, and Administration of the City of Newark, New Jersey" (November 1, 1919), pp. 318-9, Newark Public Library, New Jersey Reference Division (hereinafter referred to as Bureau of Municipal Research, N.Y., "Survey").

22. MacDougall, *Philanthropies of Newark,* pp. 22-29.

23. Bureau of Municipal Research, N.Y., "Survey," pp. 230, 301-2. My thinking in this paragraph has been guided by Sam Bass Warner Jr., *The Urban Wilderness: A History of the American City* (New York: Harper & Row, 1972), pp. 216-8.

24. For a critique of the clinic and out-patient medicine of the early twentieth century, see Warner, *Urban Wilderness,* pp. 220-2.

25. MacDougall, *Philanthropies of Newark,* p. 30; Warner, *Urban Wilderness,* pp. 220-2.

26. MacDougall, *Philanthropies of Newark,* pp. 30-31; Bureau of Municipal Research, N.Y., "Survey," pp. 330-1.

3

Board of Health

ESTABLISHMENT OF A
BACTERIOLOGICAL LABORATORY

Five horses for the production of diphtheria antitoxin awaited Dr. Richard
N. Connolly when he began work at the Newark Board of Health bacteriological laboratory on February 12, 1895. Of all the diseases that prevailed
in Newark, none was so feared as diphtheria. In treating diphtheria physicians
were confronted with the dilemma of doing nothing and watching the
child slowly choke to death or intervening with drastic therapies that
seldom worked. The disease seemed invincible.

> Strong emetics, powerful swabs and gargles, dangerous internal medi-
> cines, unsavory counterirritants applied to the throat, and last-ditch
> surgical procedures [intubations and tracheotomies] availed little.
> Not until diphtheria antitoxin was put on the market . . . did the
> slaughter of the innocents begin to diminish.[1]

Diphtheria is primarily transmitted by secretions from the nose, throat,
and lesions of infected persons and carriers. It may also be spread by
consumption of raw milk, by droplet infection, and by infected particles.
The disease occurs mainly among young children.

The first symptoms of the disease are swelling, redness, and soreness
of the throat, followed by the appearance of a yellowish false membrane
over the mucous surfaces of the throat. The spread of this membrane down
the larynx and trachea impairs breathing and, in severe cases, leads to
death from suffocation. Serious and sometimes fatal complications also
arise from the toxins produced by the diphtheria bacilli. In about 10 to 20
percent of the cases of clinical diphtheria the toxemia produces degenerative
changes in the central nervous system causing some form of paralysis,

usually in either the larynx or the palate. In other instances the heart muscles are affected, giving rise to myocarditis.[2]

The history of diphtheria is difficult to chronicle. The initial symptoms are similar to those exhibited by scarlet fever and laryngitis, and often culture tests are needed to establish a positive diagnosis. Though the disease was endemic in Europe and America throughout the first half of the nineteenth century, diphtheria was not mentioned by name in the *Transactions of the Medical Society of New Jersey* until 1861. In the decade 1850-1860 the organism responsible for diphtheria appears to have mutated and become more virulent. Thereafter diphtheria was both endemic and epidemic, and case fatality and morbidity rates skyrocketed. As diphtheria was then thought to be a "filth" disease, sanitarians tried to connect it to sewer outfalls, low, damp ground, proximity to tidewater, run-down houses, and defective drainage, all to no avail. Finally in the late nineteenth century, the microscopic agent responsible for the disease (corynebacterium diphtheriae) was found.

Antitoxin came into being after it was discovered that the pathogenesis caused by certain bacilli, notably the diphtheria and tetanus bacilli, resulted primarily from soluble poisons, known as toxins, excreted by the invading bacilli. The toxins enter into the bloodstream and attack the nervous system and other vital organs. To combat the toxins, antitoxins are produced by inoculating horses with progressively larger doses of toxins. Diphtheria antitoxin was first employed as an antidote by Emil Behring of Berlin around 1890, was subsequently administered as a prophylactic to persons who had been exposed to the disease, and since the 1920s has been used in programs of mass immunization.[3]

While Europeans such as Louis Pasteur, Robert Koch, and Behring were mainly responsible for pioneering the science of bacteriology, Americans were the first to grasp its practical applications. The multipurpose bacteriological laboratory, instrumental in the early diagnosis of disease, in the bacteriological testing of water and milk, and in the production of vaccines and serums, was an American innovation. The prototype diagnostic bacteriological laboratory was established in the New York City Department of Public Health in 1892. In the following years the laboratory was made the center of a multiple-pronged attack on diphtheria. Under the inspired leadership of Hermann M. Biggs and William H. Park, the laboratory was used to diagnose suspected cases of diphtheria, to establish the role of carriers and convalescents in transmitting the disease, and to produce antitoxin.[4]

The departures in public health made by New York City health officials came under close scrutiny in Newark. In its annual report for 1894, the Newark Board of Health argued that the creation of a bacteriological laboratory was a necessity because of the treatment it offered for diphtheria and the aid it would provide in monitoring the city's food and water supplies. Foreseeing that events in New York signaled the dawning of a new era in public health, the board was anxious that "Newark should be one of the first communities to establish . . . a laboratory and [thus] keep abreast with the advancements made in the field of preventive medicine."[5]

Dr. Richard N. Connolly of the New York City Department of Public Health was selected to run the bacteriological laboratory. An 1893 alumnus of the New York University College of Medicine with postgraduate training in bacteriology and pathology, he had worked with Drs. Park and Biggs on the production of the first batch of American-made antitoxin. The basement of the Newark City Hospital was chosen as the site of the new facility, and a resolution appropriating $5,000 for its establishment was approved by the common council. The laboratory had almost become a reality, when suddenly voices were raised against it. Mayor Julius A. Lebkuecher believed that for the city to manufacture antitoxin was socialism and therefore vetoed the resolution. In his veto message, Lebkuecher contended that: 1) the value of antitoxin had not been proven; and 2) if the drug worked, it could best be obtained commercially. The *Sunday Call* thought the cost of the laboratory extravagant and feared bacteriological laboratories might turn out to be a fad; better to spend the money on sewer construction and street cleaning, which were known disease preventives. A few persons expressed fears that the inevitable laboratory accidents would doom laboratory workers to horrible deaths and endanger the community.[6]

One day after the mayor delivered his veto, the president of the Newark Board of Health resigned. Dr. Herman Herold, who had been responsible for Connolly's appointment, now took up the fight. He warned city officials that unless the purity of the serum could be assured, public confidence in the treatment would be lost. On January 26, 1895, in a rare display of nonpartisanship three Republicans, including the Republican leader of the common council, joined forces with nine Democrats to override the mayor's veto.[7] Newark thus became one of the first cities in the United States to establish a bacteriological laboratory. Subsequently Lebkuecher sought to destroy the board of health. The attempt boomeranged and may have cost Lebkuecher his chance to win a second term in office.[8] Herold was appointed president of the board, and within a year dramatic proof of the laboratory's worth was furnished by its success in combating diphtheria.

Newark had stolen a march on other cities. A serum trust that operated in the East and the Midwest was formed in 1903. In cities which did not have bacteriological laboratories the poor were forced to pay an exorbitant price for the drug. When a bill authorizing the New Jersey State Bacteriological Laboratory to produce antitoxin was stalled in the state legislature for several years, Newark provided what relief it could to stricken communities by supplying at cost its surplus serum.[9]

The use of antitoxin in treating diphtheria produced almost theatrical effects. In some cases children said to be hovering near death were reported sitting up in bed the day after the serum was administered. The case fatality rate for those who were treated with the serum in 1895 (13 percent) was nearly half that (23 percent) for persons who went without it. Since at first the serum was used only in critical cases, its effectiveness was far greater than the figures reveal. As antitoxin was more widely prescribed, the case fatality rate for persons treated with the serum dropped sharply.[10]

Though truly a miracle-working drug, the serum had some unpleasant side effects, which impeded its acceptance. Persons sensitive to the foreign proteins contained in the drug developed serum sickness, a mild reaction characterized by skin eruptions, fever, swollen glands, and rheumatic-like pains in the joints. Acute anaphylactic shock, a much more serious problem, occurred in hypersensitive individuals within a few hours after inoculation and was sometimes fatal. Then too, there was an increase in the number of instances of postdiphtheritic paralysis as a result of the administration of the serum to persons who had already suffered irreparable damage, but who would have died had the serum not been given. In 1897 diphtheria antitoxin was resorted to in 20 percent fewer cases than in 1896.[11] Opposition to its use, wrote the Newark Board of Health in 1900, is the "most bitter . . . which the introduction of any new remedy has had to meet, with the possible exception of vaccination."[12]

With better understanding of the serum's properties, the drug gained almost total acceptance, for there was no denying its benefits. The Newark Board of Health calculated that in 1899, at a cost of $6,000, the serum had saved 321 lives. By 1916 diphtheria antitoxin was being prescribed in over 96 percent of all cases of diphtheria.[13]

As diagnostic techniques were perfected and vaccines developed, the bacteriological laboratory was employed in fighting tuberculosis, typhoid fever, malaria, syphilis, whooping cough, and rabies. Culture stations were started throughout the city, mainly in drugstores, to provide a liaison between the board of health and physicians in the Newark metropolitan area. At these depots diphtheria culture outfits, sputum jars, and vaccines were distributed, and samples for analysis were collected.[14] The scope of the bacteriological laboratory's functions can be gauged in the statistical summary below of its work for 1917.

TABLE 1

WORK OF THE NEWARK BACTERIOLOGICAL LABORATORY
FOR 1917

Diphtheria

Diphtheria cultures examined	7660
Doses of antitoxin distributed	2562

Rabies

Exposed persons given antirabic vaccine	31
Suspected animals examined	40
Culture stations maintained	50

Other Diseases

Specimens of sputa examined (tuberculosis)	3140
Blood examinations (typhoid fever and malaria)	744
Specific catarrhal infection examinations	1148
Wasserman tests	4566
Doses of typhoid fever vaccine distributed	403
Doses of pertussis (whooping cough)	
vaccine distributed	765
Water examinations	610

SOURCE: Newark Annual Reports, 1917, Board of Health, pp. 248-50.

PLATE I

DIPHTHERIA IN NEWARK, 1895-1922

(Rate per 100,000 Population)

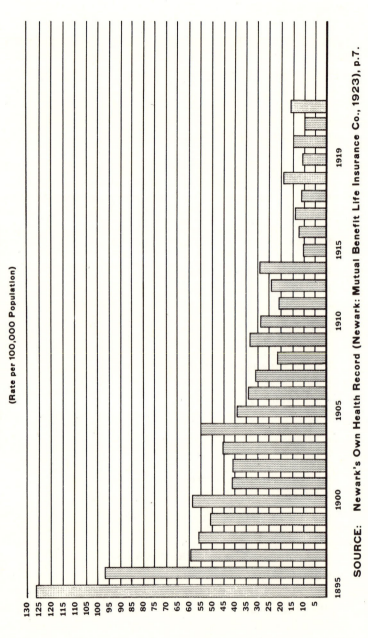

SOURCE: Newark's Own Health Record (Newark: Mutual Benefit Life Insurance Co., 1923), p.7.

28

The establishment of a bacteriological laboratory in 1895 provided a lifeline for the board of health which, until then, had been floundering in a quicksand of ineptitude, political intrigue, and public disdain. The reduction of the diphtheria mortality rate breathed new life into the board and redeemed it before the public. Furthermore, the creation of a bacteriological laboratory constitutes perhaps the single most important undertaking of the Newark Board of Health in its more than 115-year history.

ISOLATION AND DISINFECTION

As "germs" displaced "miasma," the focus of public health shifted from the control of the environment to the conquest of specific diseases. Isolation, disinfection, and immunization became the bywords for the control of infectious diseases, supplanting sanitation and cleanliness. Sanitary reform, which had been in the forefront of the Newark Board of Health's earlier endeavors, was relegated to a secondary position. In 1901 the board of health ranked the city's needs by order of importance as follows: 1) the establishment of a municipal disinfection station; 2) the building of an isolation hospital; 3) the adoption of better methods of garbage disposal; and 4) the creation of a public abattoir.[15]

As a result of the city's experience with cholera and smallpox, the Newark Board of Health had been invested with powers relating to isolation, quarantine, placarding, and disinfection many years before the advent of the germ theory of disease. But until science established the rationale for these measures, they remained in the realm of empirically derived expedients and were of little value in combating diseases with different etiologies.[16]

Physicians and private citizens alike were reticent about reporting pestilential diseases. In 1885 Newark physicians were furnished postcards and asked to report cases of scarlet fever, diphtheria, and smallpox; however, few responded.[17] Indeed, "in the majority of instances the death certificate was the first intimation received of the existence of a disease of this nature."[18]

To induce physicians to comply with the board's wishes, a variation on the stick and carrot method of persuasion was adopted. In 1886 Newark physicians were required to report all outbreaks of pestilential diseases upon penalty of a stiff fine. A state law, however, sweetened the provisions of the city ordinance by providing a $.25 payment for each case that was described. Subsequently, the list of reportable diseases was expanded. Cholera, yellow fever, and typhoid fever were added in 1888, tuberculosis in 1894, infantile paralysis in 1910, and measles, whooping cough, chicken pox, and malaria in 1912.[19]

At the suggestion of Dr. Edward E. Worl, a City Physician, a division of contagious diseases was established in 1891 within the department of health. The division, which was placed under Worl's control, was entrusted with maintaining a record of vital statistics and with finding, examining, and removing persons whose presence endangered the community. Isolating the sick was hazardous work. Not only was Worl constantly exposed to pestilential diseases, on several occasions when he attempted to remove persons to the city's hated smallpox hospital his life was threatened.[20]

Houses in which communicable diseases appeared were quarantined, placarded, and disinfected. Since the sine qua non of public health work was to prevent the sick from infecting the healthy, elaborate precautions were taken to isolate the patient along with his personal articles and any other things he might have infected. The patient was put in a separate apartment or in a little-used section of his house. A basin containing a solution of chloride of lime or carbolic acid was placed near his bed for him to spit in. The room was stripped bare of curtains, carpets, and other furnishings, and was barred to outsiders save for medical attendants and adult family members. A sheet soaked with a solution of lime, which was hung over the doorway, shielded the rest of the house and completed the cordoning of the patient's germs. These arrangements were initially supervised by the sanitary inspectors of the board of health and later by a disinfection corps created in 1894.[21] The work of the disinfection corps for a typical year, 1917, is summarized in Table 2.

Believing that domestic quarantine seldom provided adequate safeguards for either the patient or the community, Worl in 1895 was able to get two wards of twelve beds each set aside in an annex to the city hospital to treat diphtheria and scarlet fever victims. At the time, none of the city's other hospitals was admitting persons with communicable illnesses. In 1903 the annex was declared unsanitary and demolished. It was replaced by a twenty-four-bed contagious disease pavilion erected at the rear of the hospital. Since over 1,000 cases of diphtheria and scarlet fever occurred annually, only the critically ill and those who could not be isolated at home were admitted.[22]

TABLE 2

WORK OF THE NEWARK DISINFECTION CORPS FOR 1917

10,436 homes quarantined

diphtheria, scarlet fever, measles, infantile paralysis,   smallpox, epidemic

meningitis, typhoid fever (not placarded), and whooping cough (victims

required to wear arm bands).

2,968 homes disinfected

diphtheria, scarlet fever, infantile paralysis, smallpox, epidemic meningitis,

and tuberculosis.

96,939 visits and reinspections

100 funereals supervised

SOURCE: Newark Annual Reports, 1917, Board of Health, pp.206-7.

In 1894 the Newark Board of Health served notice on the common
council that it had repeatedly pleaded with it to furnish funds for the
construction of a suitable isolation hospital and consequently "any evil
resulting from the lack of a hospital for infectious diseases would rest with
it and not the Board of Health."[23] Noting that 249 children had died from
scarlet fever and diphtheria in 1894, the board warned that failure to
provide for an isolation hospital would have to be construed as "criminal
negligence" on the part of the common council.[24]

Plans to build an isolation hospital encountered the same kind of
resistance as do proposals today to maintain drug addiction centers:
everyone agrees they are necessary, but no one wants them as neighbors.
The selection of an isolation hospital site aroused heated passions. In
1900 an isolation hospital in East Orange, a suburb of Newark, was
destroyed by mob violence. When Newark tried to erect an isolation
hospital on property it owned in Livingston, angered townspeople got

the state legislature to require their consent in the project, which was
then voted down in an emotional mass meeting frequently interrupted
by cries of "pesthouse." A number of sites within Newark were appraised,
but were hastily dropped from consideration when opposition developed
from local property owners. The problem was finally "resolved" by
turning it over to the county. In 1908 the Essex County Isolation Hospital
was opened in the town of Soho.[25]

The Soho Isolation Hospital had a capacity of about 110 beds. The
number of individuals treated at the hospital varied from a little over 400
in 1917 to more than 1,000 in 1916, the year of the nation's first great
polio epidemic. About 60 percent of the persons admitted to the hospital
were from Newark.

At first the hospital was used almost exclusively for treatment of
severe cases of scarlet fever and diphtheria. Measles, chicken pox, whooping
cough, mumps, and rubella—all considered mild, almost desirable childhood
diseases, offering immunity against contracting them as an adult—were
treated at home. A tuberculosis wing for advanced cases was added to the
hospital in 1911. In 1916 the hospital was used to care for persons with
infantile paralysis, and starting in 1917 cases of cerebro-spinal meningitis
were admitted.[26]

Though vastly superior to any isolation facility hitherto established
in Essex County, the Soho hospital did not endear itself to the public. For
one thing, with the exception of mixed cases of scarlet fever and diphtheria,
the hospital lacked facilities to handle multiple infections.[27] In 1911 the
hospital refused to admit infants with diphtheria and measles sent there
by a nursery. This refusal prompted the *Newark Evening News* to exclaim
that the hospital had "failed of its purpose . . . to isolate cases that might
spread and become epidemic."[28] Beds in the tuberculosis and scarlet
fever wings were scarce, and plans for a training school for nurses were
not realized. On top of these deficiencies, there were also charges of mis-
management and political meddling.[29] "I am sorry to say," commented
Worl upon his retirement in 1923, "Newark is yet behind in these facilities
though it pays 70 percent of the expense of the county hospital. No doubt
the Soho hospital will be greatly improved."[30]

Because the most common communicable diseases of the period were
afflictions of the young, the schools became a public health battleground.
In 1885 students and teachers residing in buildings where infectious diseases
were reported were kept out of school.[31] The resulting loss of school days

was enormous, and the rule subsequently had to be modified to exclude from school only persons coming from families in which a communicable disease had actually occurred.[32]

In 1901 the boards of health and education jointly undertook the medical supervision of public school students.[33] At first the work was done by physicians engaged on a part-time basis. This proved unsatisfactory, and in 1915 a staff consisting of a large corps of nurses working under the direction of a few full-time doctors was appointed. Medical supervision was originally intended as a means of controlling the spread of infectious diseases. Other uses of the medical staff, however, were soon suggested, when large numbers of students were observed with louse-ridden clothing, dental caries, enlarged adenoids, and speech and vision impairments. In the next few years the medical supervision program was broadened to include the following duties: sanitary inspection of schools, detection of mental and physical defects, treatment of minor disorders, follow-up and referral work on ill students, and lectures and exhibits on personal hygiene.[34]

By 1911 disinfection had replaced isolation as the board of health's principal control measure for preventing epidemics.[35] The knowledge that germs cause disease led to a great upsurge in the popularity of disinfectants. It was assumed that particles of infectious material were carried great distances by air currents and were nurtured for long periods of time by persons or inanimate objects. For a while, "things" were viewed with more alarm than humans. The germ theory of disease also gave public health workers a yardstick with which to measure the effectiveness of disinfectants. Pungent but ineffective aromatics were replaced by powerful germicides. And when it was discovered that germs could not live in a toxic chemical environment, a craze for disinfection developed. During epidemics, library books, dollar bills, and even letters posted through the mails were disinfected.[36]

Until 1895 the most widely used germicide was sulphur dioxide. The gas, which was produced by burning sulphur in an iron dish, had many objectionable features. The acrid fumes made houses uninhabitable for up to twelve hours, corroded metals, made colors run, rotted fabrics, and harmed musical instruments, paintings, and other objects of art. Furthermore, though a good insecticide, sulphur dioxide was a poor germicide. In 1894 the Newark Board of Health announced that it had started construction on a steam disinfection plant.

The need for such a plant was obviated by the introduction of formaldehyde. A powerful, inexpensive, and relatively unobtrusive germicide, it was first used in Newark in 1897, and was employed for over two decades thereafter for terminal disinfection in cases of scarlet fever, diphtheria, tuberculosis, smallpox, infantile paralysis, and cerebral meningitis.[37]

Disinfectants, when properly used, play a legitimate though limited role in preventing the spread of communicable diseases. Objects needing disinfection include: 1) bodily discharges and articles soiled by them, principally bedding, clothing, toiletries, and personal effects; 2) silverware and other objects that have been mouthed; and occasionally, 3) rooms and household furnishings. Since most pathogenic microorganisms are obligate parasites of man and can survive outside the human host for only a short period of time, the usefulness of disinfectants is a function of the time and distance separating the source of infection, the patient, from the thing to be disinfected. Hence, to be effective, disinfection must be applied concurrently, during the course of the illness, rather than terminally. Terminal disinfection was first discontinued in Providence in 1912 and in several other large cities shortly thereafter.[38] Newark's health officer, however, was slow to accept the evidence and continued to employ terminal disinfection through the period under study.[39]

With the exception of tuberculosis, efforts to prevent the spread of communicable diseases by isolation and disinfection were fruitless. To the exasperation of boards of health everywhere, epidemics of measles, scarlet fever, diphtheria, and whooping cough continued unabated. Public health authorities had been overly optimistic in thinking that they could monitor the nasal and throat and bowel and bladder discharges of infected persons (from which all communicable diseases radiate). It was an impossible task. Germs were spread before officials could act or else were conveyed in unsuspected vessels. When inapparent infections outnumber clinical infections, as in infantile paralysis, when infectiousness is maximal at or shortly before the onset of symptoms, as in measles, or when there are many missed cases and carriers, as in diphtheria and scarlet fever, isolation and disinfection are not enough to prevent the spread of infection. The conquest in the last half century of such highly contagious diseases as diphtheria, scarlet fever, whooping cough, infantile paralysis, and tuberculosis has resulted not from the supervision of the sources of infection, but from the discovery of new vaccines and the introduction of chemotherapeutic drugs that render patients noninfectious.[40]

REORGANIZATION

By 1905 the Newark Board of Health had become a part of the "invisible" civil service that is the cornerstone of every modern government. But the anonymity that had come to the board was short-lived. On June 4, 1913, a report was delivered on the health department's work which would set in motion events leading to a major reorganization of the department. The report, containing scathing criticism of the organization, leadership, and activities of the health department, was made by Franz Schneider, Jr., the sanitarian of the division of surveys and exhibits of the Russell Sage Foundation, and was included in an audit of the city's governmenta' agencies made by the accounting firm of Price, Waterhouse and Company.[41]

The Newark Board of Health had failed to follow up the establishment of a bacteriological laboratory with other innovative programs. To cite one example, the board had totally overlooked the work being done in combating tuberculosis and infant mortality, though together they comprised one-third of the city's deaths. Yet the board had escaped public censure. Because of the city's declining mortality rate, the lethargy that afflicted the board had gone largely unnoticed.

A few socially minded critics had begun to fault the board for its failure to enforce the sanitary and plumbing codes in tenement districts, especially when the codes impinged upon the interests of landlords.[42] The board's inaction was not surprising, since the board was chosen from among businessmen and professionals, who shared the same class interest and outlook as the landlords. Moreover, board members were disposed to operate within the system, using their ties to persons in power to get things done.

Nominally the work of the health department was divided between the board of health and the health officer. The real power, however, lay with the board of health, which made all policy decisions. David D. Chandler, businessman and health officer of Newark for nearly thirty years, was retained by the board because of his connections with the Newark establishment and his ability to wheedle money from parsimonious city councils. The board of health was appointed by the mayor and the common council, and consisted of ten men, five of whom had to be physicians, with equal representation of the two major political parties provided for. Commented Schneider:

The present board is too large and is endowed with responsibilities which should be delegated to a competent health officer. With the recent developments in bacteriology and vital statistics, and with the establishment of great research laboratories devoted to questions of sanitation, public health science has become a decidedly technical subject, calling in its administration for expert knowledge, such as cannot be expected of the average citizen, or, for that matter, of the average physician.

An "inexpert board directing an inexpert executive certainly does not make for either a consistent or progressive policy."

The organization of the department was inefficient. The heads of its various divisions, of which there were about thirteen, exercised little authority and had to refer even trivial matters to the health officer for decision. Thus the health officer had little time "for the larger needs of health work, such as the study of health conditions in the city, [the] formulation of constructive policies, and the prosecution of vigorous campaigns." There was little coordination among divisions, even when their work was closely related, as, for example, in the case of the division of contagious diseases and the disinfection corps.

The most damaging criticism leveled against the Newark Board of Health was its failure to follow the leads of progressive health boards at a time when public health work throughout the nation was being radically expanded and transformed. Perhaps the board's most serious omission, wrote Schneider,

is the entire absence of any attempt to combat infant mortality. And this despite the fact that in 1910 over 1,200 Newark infants died before reaching the age of one. . . . It is strange indeed that the Newark department, so close to New York City—where so many valuable measures in this field have been instituted—should still entirely undervalue the importance of combating the health hazards that thus strike at the very beginnings of life and claim as a fifth of the city's entire mortality, children under one year of age.

Schneider also took the Newark Board of Health to task for its handling of milk inspection, estimating that the board was five years behind in this area. He further noted that milk inspection had only recently been undertaken by the board as a result of a newspaper exposé. These two failures

have a special significance indicating how far out of step with current progress is the policy and spirit of the department. It is clear that the department has been marking time, and giving little heed to the recent advances in public health science.

The department was also faulted for its method of compiling vital statistics, its record keeping procedures, its failure to educate the public in health matters, its administration of the municipal sanatorium, and its housing and meat and slaughterhouse inspections. The major recommendation of the report called for the appointment of a specialist in public health with "a free hand" to manage the department.

While admitting that much of the criticism was justified, both the *Newark Evening News* and the *Sunday Call* reacted angrily to Schneider's attack on the Newark Board of Health. The *News* reported that the investigation had been made at the behest of "certain powerful influences aiming to obtain domination in the department of health"[43] and that its findings would probably be accepted with reservations.

> It will require proof more definite than a general statement based on a superficial insight into affairs to convince the people of this city that this department is a moribund relic of the past, behind the times and dropping further back, and that its chief officer is inexpert and incompetent.

The *Call* was particularly miffed about the vehemence of the attack on the board's leaders, Chandler and Herold. "When criticism is made," admonished the *Call*, "it is well to look backward as well as forward." If the work of the health department had become well accepted it was because Chandler and Herold, using political, personal, and social influence ("and working for the smallest rewards"), had worked for the preceding quarter century to convince economy-minded city officials of the importance of giving the department adequate funds for its operations. Even today, added the *Call*, "you can not get an appropriation from a Mayor and thirty-two aldermen unless they like you."[44]

A year and a half passed without incident. Then in December 1914 a second bombshell was delivered, this time by the Public Welfare Committee of Essex County, an organization of civic-minded citizens which had been formed in 1911 to receive and investigate complaints about public welfare.[45] At a meeting with mayor-elect Thomas L. Raymond, three reports highly critical of the department of health, one made by the Russell Sage Foundation acting for the city, a second by the Bureau of Municipal Research of New York for the Public Welfare Committee, and a third, the report made by Price, Waterhouse and Company, were presented by the committee. The reports were in substantial agreement that the department of health was being badly mismanaged. Accounting procedures were unprofessional, they alleged, the field force was poorly supervised, and no attempt was being made to enlist the cooperation of public-spirited citizens and community organizations. The committee demanded that the department be reorganized.[46]

By now the need for reform was becoming obvious to even the board's most sympathetic supporters. Wrote the *News:*

> The alertness of former days has evidently given place to a dull spirit that prompts letting things run along in worn out grooves, and the lackadaisical feeling of time-serving has come where once energy and constructive effort prevailed.[47]

The *Call,* while still reluctant to accept the criticism in toto, conceded that the Newark Board of Health was in need of change. The partisanship and pettiness that had marked Newark political life, asserted the *Call,* was giving way. In the future everything about Newark and its government would have to be scientific, efficient, and up-to-date. Tact, diplomacy, and personal influence had achieved results "when they would not have been obtained in other ways," but if the health department was to be put on a "more scientific and less political basis," then the health officer would have to be a specialist in public health.[48] "A hundred reforms are demanded . . . new men and new ways are required."[49]

In an attempt to save itself, the Newark Board of Health instituted some new programs along the lines suggested by Schneider, but the reforms were too little and too late. In 1915 the board was turned out of office. Herold was replaced as president by Dr. William S. Disbrow, a Newark physician who had served on the board from 1895 to 1907,[50] and an interim health officer was named. State law required the new health officer to be chosen by civil service examination. The majority of the board favored the appointment of Dr. William C. Woodward, the noted former director of public health of the nation's capital, but the state civil service commission insisted that first preference be given to a New Jersey resident. In July 1915 a temporary appointment, which was made permanent in March 1916, was given to Charles Vaughn Craster. The new health department head had both an M.D. degree and a Ph.D. in public health and had served in the health departments of Glasgow, Scotland, and New York State. The health officer was made responsible for the functioning of the department, and divisions with strong executive heads were established.[51]

During the years 1915-1918 the Newark Board of Health began to display its former vigor, becoming once again an organ of progressive public health work. The supervision of the milk supply was greatly improved, and child hygiene was given a prominent place on the board's agenda.[52] Other new programs included the establishment of a division of tuberculosis, a division of venereal diseases, and a drug addiction clinic.[53] Finally, the health department started publication of a weekly bulletin. The bulletin reported the city's weekly morbidity and mortality, and contained articles of public health interest aimed principally at physicians, midwives, nurses, and school administrators.[54]

In 1919 the Bureau of Municipal Research of New York was engaged by the Newark Board of Trade to make a survey of Newark government. Commenting on the changes that had been made in the department of public health, the bureau wrote: "health service has been improved rapidly in Newark in the past few years, so that Newark stands today in the front ranks of cities as regards protection of the public health."[55] The department did not escape reproach entirely. The report found that there were still too many divisions and not enough coordination among them. A plan of reorganization was submitted, some features of which the department eventually adopted. But the report's principal recommendation, calling for the consolidation of the health department and the city hospital into a single bureau of health and hospitals, was rejected.[56]

NOTES

1. David L. Cowen, *Medicine and Health in New Jersey: A History,* Vol. XVI of *The New Jersey Historical Series,* eds. Richard M. Huber and Wheaton J. Lane (Princeton, N.J.: D. Van Nostrand Co., In., 1964), pp. 44-45. See also R. Staehlin, "Tracheotomy in Diphtheritic Croup," *Transactions of the Medical Society of New Jersey, 1866,* pp. 199-207 (hereinafter referred to as *Trans. MSNJ*), and *ARNJBH, 1890,* p. 323.

2. John Duffy, *Epidemics in Colonial America* (Baton Rouge, La.: Louisiana State University Press, 1953), pp. 113-5; Joseph A. Bell, "Diphtheria," Kenneth F. Maxcy and Milton J. Rosenau, *Preventive Medicine and Public Health,* ed. Philip E. Sartwell (9th ed., rev. and enl.;

New York: Appleton-Century-Crofts, 1965), pp. 198-9, 207; Joseph A. Vasselli, "A Pestilence Census-Taker in New Jersey," *Bulletin of the History of Medicine*, XXV (1951), 372.

3. Charles Wilcocks, *Medical Advance, Public Health, and Social Evolution* (Oxford: Pergamon Press, 1965), pp. 127-34; Richard Harrison Shryock, *The Development of Modern Medicine: An Interpretation of the Social and Scientific Factors Involved* (rev. ed.; New York: Alfred A. Knopf, 1957), pp. 297-300; George Rosen, *A History of Public Health* (New York: MD Publications, Inc., 1957), pp. 336-7.

4. Howard D. Kramer, "History of the Public Health Movement in the United States, 1850 to 1900" (Unpublished Ph.D. diss., State University of Iowa, 1942), pp. 207-9.

5. *Annual Report of the Newark Board of Health, 1894*, p. 37.

6. *Newark Evening News*, Jan. 10, 12, 1895, Jan. 20, 1922, March 25, 1953; *Sunday Call*, Jan. 20, 27, 1895, March 29, 1936.

7. *Newark Evening News*, Jan. 10, 12, 1895, Jan. 20, 1922.

8. *Sunday Call*, January 27, 1895; *Newark Evening News*, Jan. 28, 1895; *New Jersey Review of Charities and Corrections*, III (1904), 19 (hereinafter referred to as *NJRCC*).

9. *NJRCC*, III (1904), 208-9, V (1906), 148-9, VII (1908), 93; *Sunday Call*, Jan. 17, 1904.

10. *Sunday Call*, March 29, 1936; H.C.H. Herold, "Newark's Diphtheria Antitoxin Plant—Its Results and Costs," *Annual Report of the Newark Board of Health, 1900*, pp. 29-33; *Newark Annual Reports, 1915, Board of Health*, p. 1021.

11. Rosenau, *Preventive Medicine*, 1st ed., p. 152, 6th ed., pp. 70, 72; Bell, "Diphtheria," p. 200.

12. *Annual Report of the Board of Health, 1900*, p. 49.

13. Herold, "Newark's Diphtheria Antitoxin Plant," p. 36; *Newark Annual Reports, 1916, Board of Health*, p. 1236.

14. *Newark Annual Reports, 1915, Board of Health*, p. 1021.

15. *Newark Annual Reports, 1901, Board of Health*, p. 14.

16. Rosenau, *Preventive Medicine*, 6th ed., pp. 669-75.

17. *Newark Annual Reports, 1885, Board of Health*, pp. 609-10; *1886, Board of Health*, pp. 587-8.

18. *Newark Annual Reports, 1887, Board of Health*, p. 484.

19. *Newark Annual Reports, 1882, Board of Health*, p. 426, *1886*, pp. 587-8; New Jersey, *Legislative Acts* (1886), p. 293; Newark, *The Sanitary Code Adopted by the Board of Health of the City of Newark, N.J., June 1888*, p. 70.

20. *Sunday Call*, Jan. 21, 1923; *Newark Evening News*, October 30,

1942; Bureau of Municipal Research, N.Y., "Survey," p. 253.

21. *Newark Annual Reports, 1881, Board of Health*, p. 411, *1917*, pp. 206-7; *Annual Report of the Board of Health, 1894*, pp. 25-26.

22. *Sunday Call*, March 10, 1895, Jan. 21, 1923; *Newark Evening News*, Oct. 1, 1903; A.W. MacDougall, *The Philanthropies of Newark, New Jersey: A Descriptive Directory* (n.p. 1916), pp. 25-30; Bureau of Municipal Research, N.Y., "Survey," p. 297.

23. *Annual Report of the Board of Health, 1894*, p. 24. See also *Newark Annual Reports, 1886, Board of Health*, pp. 588-9; *Annual Report of the Board of Health, 1888*, p. 10, *1889*, p. 11.

24. *Annual Report of the Board of Health, 1894*, pp. 24-25.

25. *Newark Evening News*, March 27, April 20, 24, 1901; *Annual Report of the Board of Health, 1902*, p. 36; New Jersey, *Legislative Acts* (1903), pp. 155, 238-40; Essex County, *Report of the Isolation Hospital, 1908-1909*, p. 327.

26. Essex County, *Report of the Isolation Hospital, 1908-1909*, p. 324, *1909-1910*, pp. 334-5, 340, *1910-1911*, p. 623; *1916-1917*, p. 381, *1918*, p. 235.

27. Essex County, *Report of the Isolation Hospital, 1912-1913*, p. 391.

28. *Newark Evening News*, April 21, 26, 1911.

29. Essex County, *Report of the Isolation Hospital, 1913-1914*, pp. 311, 336, *1916-1917*, p. 381; *NJRCC*, VII (1908), 165-6.

30. *Sunday Call*, Jan. 21, 1923.

31. *Annual Report of the Board of Education, 1885*, p. 212. Subsequently a certificate from the board of health was required for all but minor infectious diseases. *Annual Report of the Board of Education, 1901*, p. 241, *1909*, p. 270.

32. *Annual Report of the Board of Education, 1912*, pp. 214-5, *1913*, pp. 142-3.

33. *Annual Report of the Board of Health, 1899*, pp. 17-19; *Annual Report of the Board of Education, 1900*, pp. 56-57, *1902*, p. 303, *1904*, pp. 302-4, *1905*, pp. 162-3. In 1909 the board of education assumed sole responsibility for the work. *Annual Report of the Board of Education, 1909*, p. 60.

34. *Annual Report of the Board of Education, 1902*, pp. 303, 390, *1909*, p. 61, *1912*, p. 218, *1915*, p. 242, *1916*, p. 245; MacDougall, *Philanthropies of Newark*, p. 68.

35. J. Wilmer Kennedy, *Newark in the Public Schools of Newark: A Course of Study on Newark, its Geography, Civics, and History, with Biographical Sketches and a Reference Index* (Newark: Newark Board of Education, 1911), p. 49.

36. Wilson G. Smillie, *Public Health, Its Promise for the Future: A Chronicle of the Development of Public Health in the United States, 1607-1914* (New York: The Macmillan Co., 1955), pp. 363-8.

37. Rosenau, *Preventive Medicine*, 6th ed., p. 1392; *Annual Report of the Newark Board of Health, 1894*, pp. 25-29; *1897*, pp. 36-38; *Newark Annual Reports, 1917, Board of Health*, pp. 206-7; Smillie, *Public Health, Its Promise for the Future*, p. 364.

38. Rosenau, *Preventive Medicine*, 6th ed., pp. 1379-81; Bureau of Municipal Research, N.Y., "Survey," p. 255.

39. *Newark Evening News*, July 30, 1915; Bureau of Municipal Research, N.Y., "Survey," pp. 255-7; Smillie, *Public Health, Its Promise for the Future*, pp. 367-8; Rosenau, *Preventive Medicine*, 6th ed., pp. 1379-9

40. Rosenau, *Preventive Medicine*, 5th ed., pp. 527-8; 6th ed., pp. 956-7; Paul M. Denson and Winston H. Price, "General Epidemiology of Infections," Rosenau, *Preventive Medicine*, 9th ed., p. 89.

41. Though the actual report could not be located, large sections of it were quoted in the *Newark Evening News*. The passages below are based on the account found in the *Newark Evening News*.

42. See Chapter 11.

43. A political struggle may have been shaping up between Herold and the city's Democratic administration. Herold was prominent in local Republican circles. Before his death in 1922, he was, at various times, a candidate for mayor of Newark and president of the Essex County Republican Society. *Newark Evening News*, Jan. 20, 1922.

44. *Sunday Call*, June 8, 1913.

45. *NJRCC*, IX, No. 10 (Oct. 1911), 13-14.

46. *Newark Evening News*, Dec. 12, 1914. The reports have not been found.

47. Ibid., Dec. 15, 1914.

48. *Sunday Call*, Dec. 20, 1914.

49. Ibid., Feb. 14, 1915.

50. *Newark Evening News*, Feb. 19, 1915.

51. Ibid., Feb. 19, Dec. 23, 1915, Dec. 9, 1953.

52. Below, chaps. VII and VIII.

53. *Newark Annual Reports, Board of Health, 1918*, pp. 163, 188.

54. Newark, Department of Public Health, *Weekly Bulletin*, N.S., Vol. I, No. 1 (June 12-19, 1915). Efforts to publish a periodical before 1915 proved abortive.

55. Bureau of Municipal Research, N.Y., "Survey," p. 231.

56. Ibid., pp. 231-69.

PLATE II   ORGANIZATION OF THE NEWARK DEPARTMENT OF HEALTH, 1919

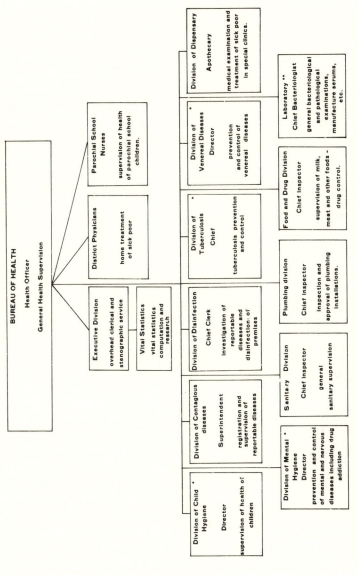

SOURCE: Bureau of Municipal Research, N.Y., "Survey," p.232.

* These divisions work in close cooperation with the dispensary service.
** Located at City Hospital

43

4

Water Supply

TYPHOID FEVER EPIDEMICS OF 1898 AND 1899

A twenty-year period in which typhoid fever, dysentery, and other water-borne diseases had plagued Newark came to an end in 1892 when the city signed a contract with the East Jersey Water Company for a supply of pure mountain water from the Pequannock River. But while the worst was over, Newark was not out of the woods yet. For one thing the city had miscalculated its immediate water needs and in 1899 would again have to drink from the Passaic River with disastrous results. The Pequannock watershed would have to be protected against pollution. It would be necessary to institute sanitary inspections, to abate nuisances, and to acquire property in the area. Such measures would safeguard the water supply against the most obvious and dangerous nuisances, but would not eliminate the risk of contamination through accident. To be on guard against all eventualities, Newark officials would begin chemical treatment and bacteriological testing of the water supply. And by the time the Pequannock safety was assured, it would be necessary to seek an additional water supply.

Foresight had been shown in contracting for a water supply three and one-half times in excess of the community's existing water requirements. Newark's population had increased by about one-third in each of the three preceding decades and would grow even faster in the years 1892-1918. As living standards rose and indoor plumbing became commonplace, per capita consumption of water increased sharply. In 1870 an average of 36 gallons per capita was consumed daily; by 1890, the per capita average was about 77.4 gallons.[1] The continuing industrial boom along with the development of heavy manufacturing in Newark added greatly to the demand. Industries had a seemingly insatiable thirst and were Newark's largest consumers of water.[2]

Tragically, the wisdom displayed by the municipal fathers in securing
a large water supply was offset by a false economy. To save money
Newark had agreed to use only 27.5 million gallons of water daily
until 1900 (when the full 50-million-gallon supply would become available).
Daily consumption of water in 1890 was a little over 14 million gallons.[3]
Thereafter, it increased an average of about 2 million gallons each year,
reaching 27.4 million gallons by 1898.[4] These figures only indicate
average daily usage. On very hot days, and on very cold days when faucets
were turned on to prevent pipes from freezing, consumption climbed
precipitately. As the city lacked adequate reservoir facilities to store water
not used during periods of low consumption, any prolonged period of
adverse weather dangerously lowered the level of water in the reservoirs.[5]

The subject of a supplementary water supply for emergency use was
first broached in 1896 by Harrison Van Duyne, the president of the Board
of Street and Water Commissioners,[6] in a letter to the East Jersey Water
Company.[7] At the time the city and the water company were engaged
in a heated controversy. The contract required the company to build
reservoirs and conduits capable of supplying Newark with 50 million
gallons of water per day. In dispute was a reservoir, Canistear Reservoir,
and a third pipeline which the city wanted built.[8] Municipal officials
were confident that the courts would uphold their claims when the contract
expired in 1900. Also they had a trump card to play which they believed
would enable them to wait out the water company should demand exceed
27.5 million gallons before 1900, as seemed likely. In 1896 the pumping
machinery at the old Belleville (Passaic River) waterworks had been
reactivated. Should there be a water crisis, the city fathers intended to
use the pumps to suck up water trapped in underground strata in the
vicinity of the Belleville filtration basins and nearby privately owned
driven wells, whose water the city had considered using in 1879. Under
these circumstances meaningful negotiations were impossible.[9]

The city's calculations allowed no margin for error. The danger of
using Passaic River water, should the need arise, was underscored by
events during the summer and fall of 1898. Through the agency of a
leaky valve, water from the Passaic River found its way into the main
Pequannock pipeline. During the months of August, September, and
October there were 126 cases of typhoid fever, nearly four times the
number which had occurred during the same months of the previous
year.[10] Moreover, bacteriological examination revealed that the water in

the Belleville basins was contaminated, probably by seepage from the Passaic River.[11] The city had lost its gamble.

As an alternative to obtaining an additional water supply, Van Duyne now proposed that the introduction of water meters be accelerated. About 3.4 million gallons, or 15 percent of the water supply, was metered. Metering was opposed by the saloons, in which Newark was rich, and by the other business establishments that paid flat water fees. Though these firms consumed 65 percent of the supply, they accounted for only 17.1 percent of the income derived from water receipts. "It is the saloon-keeper," wrote the *Sunday Call*, "that the politician in the Board of Works is afraid of."[12] Party rivalries also entered into the fray. Starting in 1894, the officials of the board of street and water commissioners were popularly elected.[13] Van Duyne and the other Republicans who sat on the board favored the introduction of meters, whereas the Democrats, who were in the majority, were partisan toward wells.[14]

In November 1898 new driven wells were sunk at the Belleville pumping station in the hope of tripling the existing yield of about 2 million gallons.[15] In July 1898 bargaining began with the East Jersey Water Company. The company had the city over a barrel. In exchange for an emergency water supply the company asked that Newark pay the construction costs of a third aqueduct to carry the additional water (a tacit admission of Newark's position in its dispute with the company over the need for a third pipeline) and also allow use of the surplus waters that would become available when final payment was made on the contract in 1900.[16] The reaction of the city was best summed up in an editorial of the *Sunday Call* which warned that the "game" was one that two could play, and that Newark's turn at bat was coming.[17] The impasse would lead to disaster.

By 1899 the reservoirs were nearly depleted. On January 11 a leather tannery was gutted by fire because of lack of sufficient pressure in the mains. Fire insurance companies started canceling policies and would not issue new ones.[18] The worst was yet to come. Midway through February a severe storm, the second worst of its kind in fifty years, lashed Newark with gale winds, heavy snows, and freezing cold. In many buildings faucets were turned on to prevent pipes from freezing. As the water level in the reservoirs fell, so, correspondingly, did the pressure in the distributing system. In several sections of Newark there was no water above the second floor. Citizens who could not obtain water bombarded the board of works by messenger and phone calls with appeals for relief. Because of public pressure and the fire hazard to the city, beginning on

February 13 and lasting until February 18, Passaic River water was mixed with the Pequannock supply. Residents were warned to boil the water, which upon analysis was found to be grossly contaminated. During the months of March, April, and May there were 395 cases and 50 deaths from typhoid fever, plus "numerous cases" of violent diarrhea and dysentery, 58 of which were fatal.[19] The lower sections of Newark, including all of the "Down Neck" area, took the heaviest toll, there being "but few homes, particularly among those who were unable to purchase special brands of drinking water, where it did not find victims."[20]

In February 1899 plans were announced for the construction of a large storage reservoir,[21] and in April the city disclosed that it would purchase a 5-million-gallon supply of artesian well water from wells to be dug at the Belleville pumping station. The city's plan to revive the discredited driven well proposal was angrily denounced in many quarters as a scheme to enrich a few politically influential businessmen at the taxpayer's expense. Bacteriological examination of water taken from the driven wells at Belleville on February 15 had shown a high bacteria count plus the presence of colon bacilli, and it was feared the new water supply would be similarly contaminated. With the support of the Newark Board of Trade, four prominent citizens went to court in an unsuccessful effort to block the project. The *Sunday Call* termed it a "job" put forth by the Democratic bosses. In fact, in both the board of works and the common council the measure had been secured by the partisan votes of lame duck Democratic majorities.[22] As security against the failure of the wells, the city also signed a contract with the East Jersey Water Company for an additional supply of water—though on far better terms than had been offered the previous year.[23] Finally, in May, the board of works, which was now under Republican control, ordered an extensive metering of the water supply. The plumbing repairs made by homeowners, who suddenly became attentive to water loss from leaks and drips, plus the more frugal consumption of water brought about by metering, netted the city a daily saving of nearly 6 million gallons of water.[24] Never again would Newarkers drink the filthy waters of the Passaic River.

PROTECTION OF THE PEQUANNOCK WATER SUPPLY

The city authorities had chosen wisely in selecting the Pequannock for Newark's water supply. The drainage area tributary to the intake reservoir, about sixty-two square miles in area, is a natural wilderness: mountainous, heavily forested, and lightly populated.[25] Still, even the purest water can be defiled. An inspection of the area in 1893 disclosed the existence of ninety-seven sources of actual or possible contamination: sixty-six from privies located near streams, including five that were either built over streams or drained into them by sewers, and thirty-one from barns and pigsties.[26] Newark's health officer warned that "under the present conditions, should typhoid fever or cholera occur in the Pequannock region, the germs of these diseases might readily find their way into the water, and would in consequence prove a source of great danger to this community."[27]

The board of works, which had the responsibility of protecting the watershed, made only sporadic efforts to guard the area from pollution. Reports of nuisances were investigated and impromptu sanitary inspections were made of the Pequannock River and its tributaries, but no regular plan of inspection existed. The board did take one action to prevent future recurrences of nuisances, which was to build new privy vaults for the inhabitants of the region whenever old vaults, because of their location or poor construction, threatened to pollute the streams.[28]

The precautions exercised by the board of works were inadequate. In 1897 the board of health, which had started making monthly analyses of the water supply, reported the presence of colon bacilli in their samples, indicating fecal contamination. Complaints were also received that the water was brackish. An inquiry conducted by the board of health turned up some embarrassing facts. The city had hired a man to prevent squatters from moving into municipally owned buildings in the watershed region. A believer in the free enterprise system, the man had rented the property to laborers and had turned the house that the city allowed him to occupy into a saloon.

The source of pollution was traced to Brown's Hotel at Newfoundland, just above the intake reservoir. Normally the sewage from the hotel was drained onto a sandy plot of ground where it was treated. Heavy rains, however, had transformed a nearby brook into a rampaging stream which had swept down through the existing outdoor sanitary facilities at the hotel, carrying off with it the hotel's sewage.[29] The *Sunday Call* commented that "while the area from which the water is drawn is sparsely populated, and it would be easy to prevent contamination, lack of supervision might produce disaster in the event of a typhoid outbreak in the region."[30]

The responsibility for protecting Newark's water supply was divided between the board of health, which had the task of looking after the health of the city, and the board of works, which had the job of seeing that the East Jersey Water Company supplied "good and wholesome" water as stipulated in the contract. Unfortunately, the close cooperation of the boards necessitated by this division of responsibility did not exist. Results of investigations and laboratory tests conducted by one board were not made known to the other. Difficulties also arose from the fact that the East Jersey Water Company retained legal title to the waterworks until 1900. It was the policy of the boards to rely upon the company to bring suit against polluters. In arguing that the company and the city had an "identity of interests" in keeping the Pequannock clean, the boards failed to recognize that the company's stake in pure water was negligible and indirect, whereas to the citizens of Newark pure water was a matter of life and death.[31]

Relations between the board of works and the board of health reached their nadir during the typhoid fever epidemic of 1898. Initially, the board of health suspected that the disease had been brought to Newark by returning veterans of the Spanish-American War. Subsequently, it examined the milk and water supplies and found that the water in the basins at Belleville was contaminated. The board of health thereupon adopted a resolution calling for the abandonment of both the water in the basins and the water in the nearby driven wells. The board of works refused to comply with the order on the grounds that the board of health had tested the water of mixed samples and had not examined samples taken solely from the driven wells. Moreover, the board of works accused the board of health of trying to throw up a smokescreen to distract attention from its failure to rid the Pequannock watershed of nuisances. Though further tests revealed that the water from the driven wells was safe, the conduct of the board of works during the epidemic did it little credit, as it had known for some time that the city's main source of water supply was being contaminated by a leaky valve and had kept this knowledge from the board of health.[32]

Beginning about the time that the city gained title to the waterworks (1900), the two boards began to act in greater harmony. Why after years of quarreling they suddenly became reconciled is unclear. Perhaps the explanation for their rapprochement lay in their sense of increased responsibilities brought on by city ownership of the waterworks. At any rate, employees of the board of health were detailed to assist the board of works in making surveys of the watershed and in collecting samples. A system of regular sanitary examination of the Pequannock Valley was initiated in which the watershed was divided into six districts, each of which was inspected weekly.[33]

In making its annual report for 1894, the board of health had expressed the fear that the Pequannock region would be developed as a summer resort area and its waterways tapped, or worse, turned into sewers. To forestall this possibility, legislation was passed giving Newark the right to build and maintain waterworks and sewerage for the Pequannock region. Newark officials were particularly concerned about the danger from Newfoundland, the largest town in the watershed area, and were prepared to spend upwards of $100,000 in the community on sewerage, water mains, and other capital improvements. But opposition from Newfoundland residents, who resented Newark's intrusion into the town's affairs, forced the city to find another way of protecting the watershed.[34] Starting about 1906 the city began acquiring property in the Pequannock watershed and over the next 12 years spent upwards of $11.5 million on land purchases. By 1918 the city had come into possession of about 70 percent of the catchment area, including all of the land bordering the streams and the reservoirs.[35]

Protection of the water supply was strengthened in other ways as well. Daily bacteriological examinations of the water in city reservoirs and house faucets monitored the purity of the water supply and provided a red alert in case of pollution. The testing was first done by the board of health and later was also undertaken by the water department of the board of works. After discovering that the growth of algae in the reservoirs was causing tap water to become cloudy and "fishy," the water supply was regularly treated with copper sulphate. In 1913 a chlorine disinfection plant was built for emergency use. At the request of the Newark Board of Health, the state board of health was authorized to close the toilets on trains when they passed through the Pequannock watershed. A large storage basin, Cedar Grove Reservoir, with excellent facilities for aeration, clarification, and sedimentation, was constructed. A program of reforestation was started to prevent soil erosion and excess water runoff. Between 1908 and 1910 some 250,000 white ash, spruce, and pine trees were planted. In 1912 a model village, Macopin, was built below the intake reservoir to relocate all native residents living on city-owned property in the area, who in 1912 numbered some 900 persons.[36]

WANAQUE WATERWORKS

With average daily consumption increasing at the rate of nearly 2 million gallons per year, even a 50-million-gallon supply would soon become insufficient. Newark officials, led by Morris R. Sherrerd, the chief engineer of the water department, wanted to tap the water of the Wanaque River,[37] one of the upper tributaries of the Passaic River. When Paterson and other cities objected that Newark would gain a monopoly of the area's water resources, the matter was turned over to a state commission that had been created in 1907 to consider problems of flood control and water supply.

Studies made by the state water supply commission led to plans for state financing of a Wanaque waterworks project to provide water for the communities in the northern New Jersey metropolitan area. State voters, however, rejected an enabling bond issue, and it became necessary to shift the burden of financing the waterworks from the state to the local communities that would benefit from it. The project was moved one step closer to completion in 1916 with the creation of the Northern Jersey District Water Supply Commission to coordinate and oversee the efforts of the communities under its jurisdiction in developing a joint waterworks.

The statute establishing the Northern Jersey District Water Supply Commission provided that contracts be entered into between it and the participating municipalities. Newark had been ready for some time to go ahead with the development of the waterworks and in the next two years helped underwrite the cost of surveys and other preliminary work. But other communities procrastinated, and the project might have fallen through had not Newark agreed to finance the entire cost of construction, estimated at $9 million, until such time as the foot-dragging communities agreed to join in the undertaking. A contract for the development of a 50-million-gallon daily supply (later expanded to 100 million) was signed in 1918. Largely through the diplomacy of Newark mayor Thomas L. Raymond, the communities that had been reluctant to participate were persuaded to take part in the venture. Work was begun on the Wanaque waterworks in 1920, and the supply was put in service in 1930.

NOTES

1. New Jersey, *Legislative Documents* (1884), Vol. II, Doc. 40, *Report of the Commissioners of State Water Supply of New Jersey, March 1884,*

Supplementary Report, p. 9; U.S. Bureau of the Census, *Eleventh Census of the United States, 1890: Report on Vital and Social Statistics,* II, 3.

2. Samuel Harry Popper, "Newark, N.J., 1870-1910: Chapters in the Evolution of an American Metropolis" (Unpublished Ph.D. diss., New York University, 1952), pp. 17-19.

3. U.S., Bureau of the Census, *Eleventh Census of the United States, 1890: Report on Vital and Social Statistics,* II, 3.

4. *Newark Annual Reports, 1898, Board of Street and Water Commissioners, p. 99.*

5. Newark, *Report* [of the Engineer of the Water Department] *to the Board of Street and Water Commissioners of the City of Newark, N.J., February 28, 1894* (n.p., 1894), pp. 11-16.

6. In 1891, the New Jersey legislature adopted a bill authorizing cities of the first class to create boards with law-making powers to administer various city services. The board of street and water commissioners was given control over water supply, sewers, and waste disposal. Popper, "Newark," pp. 280-3.

7. *Sunday Call,* January 26, 1896.

8. Ibid.; *Newark Evening News,* April 14, 1936.

9. *Sunday Call,* January 26, 1896; *Newark Annual Reports, 1896, Board of Street and Water Commissioners,* p. 11.

10. William S. Disbrow, "A Municipal Molech," *Trans. MSNJ, 1899,* pp. 273-4; H.C.H. Herold, "Report on Typhoid Fever, Newark, New Jersey: 1898-1899," *Reports and Papers of the American Public Health Association,* XXV (1899), 173-74; *Annual Report of the Board of Health, 1898,* pp. 40, 99, 107; *Newark Evening News,* Oct. 15, 1898.

11. *Newark Evening News,* Oct. 6, 7, 1898.

12. *Sunday Call,* Aug. 7, 1898.

13. Popper, "Newark," pp. 281-2.

14. *Newark Evening News,* November 10, 1898, May 2, 1899.

15. Ibid., Nov. 10, 1898.

16. Ibid., Sept. 15, 1898, Feb. 14, 1899; *Sunday Call,* Sept. 18, 1898.

17. *Sunday Call,* Sept. 18, 1898.

18. *Newark Evening News,* Jan. 11, 1899.

19. Disbrow, "A Municipal Molech," pp. 275-78; Herold, "Report on Typhoid Fever," pp. 173-6; *Annual Report of the Board of Health, 1899,* pp. 35-40; *Newark Evening News,* Feb. 11, 13, March 8, 1899; *Newark Annual Reports, 1898, Board of Street and Water Commissioners,* pp. 98-99. (The report of the water department for 1898 was sent to the printer late. Thus the chief engineer of the department was able to include the events of February 1899 in his report for 1898.)

20. Disbrow, "A Municipal Molech," p. 275.

21. *Newark Evening News,* Feb. 19, 1899.

22. *Sunday Call,* April 16, 23, 30, 1899; *Newark Evening News,* April 14, 1899; *Annual Report of the Board of Health, 1899,* pp. 58, 72. The wells were built but were resorted to only once for a period of one day. After 1900 the pumps were maintained on a standby emergency basis. *Newark Annual Reports, 1900, Board of Street and Water Commissioners,* p. 6.

23. *Newark Evening News,* April 14, 24, 1899.

24. Ibid., May 2, 1899; *Newark Annual Reports, 1899, Board of Street and Water Commissioners,* pp. 94-97.

25. *Sunday Call,* May 12, 1912; *ARNJBH, 1912,* p. 386. The Pequannock watershed is located thirty-five miles northwest of Newark in Morris, Passaic, and Sussex counties.

26. *Annual Report of the Board of Health, 1894,* pp. 39-43; Charles Lehlbach, "The Newark Water Supply," *ARNJBH, 1893,* pp. 55-59.

27. Lehlbach, "Newark Water Supply," p. 57.

28. *Sunday Call,* May 12, 1912.

29. Ibid., Aug. 15, 22, 1897, March 29, 1936.

30. Ibid., Aug. 15, 1897.

31. *Newark Evening News,* Feb. 3, Sept. 23, 1899; *Sunday Call,* Aug. 15, 1897, Aug. 20, 1899.

32. *Newark Evening News,* Sept. 16, 21, 23, Oct. 6, 7, 15, 1898.

33. *Sunday Call,* May 12, 1912; *Newark Evening News,* August 15, 1899; *Newark Annual Reports, 1901, Board of Street and Water Commissioners,* p. 8, *1902, Board of Health,* p. 468.

34. *Annual Report of the Board of Health, 1894,* pp. 39-43; *Sunday Call,* May 12, 1912; *Newark Annual Reports, 1893, Board of Street and Water Commissioners,* p. 49.

35. *Sunday Call,* May 12, 1912; *Newark Evening News,* May 2, 1908; *Newark Annual Reports, 1912, Board of Health,* p. 387; Bureau of Municipal Research, N.Y., "Survey," p. 563.

36. *Newark Annual Reports, 1908, Board of Street and Water Commissioners,* pp. 459-60; *ARNJBH, 1912,* pp. 386-8, *1913,* p. 409; *Sunday Call,* May 12, 1912; Bureau of Municipal Research, N.Y., "Survey," p. 563.

37. The story of the Wanaque Project is based primarily upon N.J., *North Jersey District Water Supply Commission Report, 1916-1925* (n.p., n.d.), pp. 3-6, 226-7. Also used were: *Sunday Call,* May 12, 1912, March 29, 1936; *Newark Evening News,* April 14, 1936; Arthur H. Pratt, *The Wanaque Water-Works Project,* reprinted from the *Journal of the New England Water Works Association,* Vol. XLIV, No. 3 (Sept. 1930), pp. 387-91; *Newark Annual Reports, 1918, Board of Street and Water Commissioners,* p. 1047; N.J., Water Supply Commission, *Annual Report, 1908,* pp. 5-7, *1910,* pp. 3-4, 10; James W. Costello, "Water Supply of the City of Newark," *Journal of Industry and Finance,* XII (Feb. 1938), 27.

5

Passaic Valley Trunk Sewer

Before it became hopelessly polluted, the Passaic River was a treasured recreational retreat for Newarkers. The river was a paradise for both commercial and noncommercial fishermen; crabs and shrimp were easily scooped up in its creeks and inlets, while in midstream lines and nets brought up perch, pickerel, shad, smelt, and bass. In the better restaurants, gourmets feasted on Passaic River shad and smelt. The river was one of the biggest shad fishing areas in the East and often attracted fishing parties from New York and Brooklyn, whose business provided a source of income for local boat owners, fishing guides, and merchants.[1]

The piers that lined the watercourse invited swimmers. Diving posed little hazard because objects could be seen on the bottom at a depth of ten to fifteen feet. A little further upstream, the tree-shaded estates of many of Newark's most prominent families bordered the river. Much of the city's social life revolved around the waterway. Exclusive clubs held regattas, and the river was used extensively for canoeing and picnicking. Undoubtedly, the idyllic scenery was a catalyst in many courtships. Private citizens also utilized the river as an artery of transportation. Families living along its banks visited one another by boat, and commuters rowed to the eastern shore to catch the coach that took them to the Hudson ferry.[2]

Boat-racing became a popular pastime of the American people after the Civil War. In the winter of 1874-1875 the boat clubs along the Passaic organized the Passaic River Amateur Rowing Association, which shortly thereafter held races twice a year, on July 4 and on Memorial Day. The events ran from dawn to dusk and attracted thousands of onlookers who braved the precarious perches of small boats and crowded grandstands to cheer their favorite crews to victory.[3] Indeed, rowers rivaled baseball players in popularity.[4] In this and in countless other ways, the river afforded an opportunity to escape, if only briefly, from the pressures and discomforts of urban living, and to look upon and delight in nature's wonders

For reasons of geography, the Passaic River was not long destined to retain its pristine beauty. The Passaic rises in the hills of Somerset County and flows northerly and easterly until it reaches Paterson. Up to this point it washes a largely agricultural area and is relatively free of contamination. At Paterson, however, the character of the river changes abruptly. The river now turns south passing through the most highly developed section of New Jersey, for which it is the natural drainage outlet, until it reaches Newark Bay, a scant twenty-two miles distant. As the tempo of urbanization and industrialization gained momentum after the Civil War, the volume of untreated sewage and industrial wastes poured into the Passaic increased until the waterway had the characteristics of an open sewer.[5] Its condition first drew the attention of the communities dependent upon it for their water supply. During the 1880s a concerted but futile effort was made by Newark and Jersey City to safeguard the river against pollution.[6] As cities in quest of a better water supply abandoned the Passaic River for the sweet waters of the upper Passaic watershed, the freshwater flow of the Passaic decreased and the condition of the river grew worse. By 1908 the Passaic's daily dry-weather flow had dropped from 85 million gallons to scarcely 35 million gallons.[7]

The fishing industry died and the stately homes and estates along the river were converted into junkyards and smoke-belching factories. Industrialization accelerated the destruction of the river as manufacturers began spewing their wastes into it. The shortsightedness of this cavalier disregard for a natural resource became apparent during periods of hot weather, when the river emitted a stench so overpowering that factories were forced to stop production. Floating debris, murky water, and raw sewage made swimming unsafe, and the bathhouses on the river had to be closed. The pleasure craft that had dotted the river were replaced by decaying boat hulks, and in 1901 the regattas came to an end.[8] The *Newark Evening News* commented that

> the property, [the] health, and even the lives of more people are menaced by the sewage-laden water than by any other agency which the residents of the affected district have had to deal with. Without exaggeration it may be said that 500,000 persons are, directly, or indirectly, exposed to the disease-breeding-effluvium and noxious odors of the river.[9]

A long drought during the summer of 1894 turned the Passaic River into a cesspool. Houses adjacent to the Passaic River below Paterson were deserted, and in Newark the river's stench caused an epidemic of nose-holding and nausea.[10] The distress caused by the river's pollution led the New Jersey Board of Health to submit two relief bills to the legislature that year: one proposing the appointment of a commission to consider a general system of drainage for the Passaic River Valley; and the other investing the board of health with the power to plan sewer systems to prevent the further pollution of any river used for drinking. When both bills failed, the board changed its tactics and attempted to get the legislature's attention by drumming up public protests about the river's foul condition.

At a meeting of the boards of health of the lower Passaic River Valley called by the state board of health in 1895, reports were read detailing the blight, the increased sickness, the nauseating odors, and the economic losses brought on by the river's pollution.[11] Pressure was also applied by the Newark Board of Trade and the communities bordering the river, leading in 1896 to the establishment of a state investigatory commission.[12] After exhaustive study of the various methods of sewage disposal in the United States and Europe, the commission recommended the construction of a trunk sewer along the course of the Passaic River below Paterson to intercept and carry the sewage of the valley into Newark Bay.

The state investigatory commission proposed the Newark Bay outlet with reservations. From a hydrographic standpoint Newark Bay is poorly suited for diluting and oxidizing sewage. The bay, a landlocked, rectangular tidal basin six miles long and about one and one-third miles wide, is very shallow and has a cross section resembling a skimming dish. Over large areas the average depth at low waters is between two and three feet. The bay's outlets are meager and the currents weak. The net ebb flow seaward measures only one-nineteenth part of the tidal prism. Freshwater and saltwater inflow into the basin are small. The few good channels for carrying off sewage are poorly located. In summer the temperature of the water is high, a condition favoring bacterial growth and decomposition. The committee endorsed the Newark Bay outlet because of the lower construction costs afforded by a nearby outfall. It counseled, however, that should it become necessary to purify the sewage before its discharge into Newark Bay, the best solution would be to emit raw sewage into upper New York Bay. Communities located on Newark Bay, and especially Bayonne, understandably feared their commerce and health would be threatened by the proposed outlet and lodged a strong protest against the scheme. The high costs that were contemplated scared off other communities and the project was shelved.[13]

But concerned citizens refused to allow the issue to die. Newark, which suffered more than other communities because of the action of the tide, was especially active in the campaign to purify the river. The city's Board of Trade intensified its lobbying activities, while local newspapers kept the subject constantly before the public. Persons living, owning property, or engaged in business along the river instituted court actions to enjoin municipalities from polluting the river. In 1898 a second state commission endorsed the trunk sewer plan. Unwilling to commit itself on this politically sensitive subject, the legislature then turned the matter over to still a third body, the State Sewerage Commission, a permanent commission established in 1899 to protect all the potable waters of the state.[14]

A provision of the law establishing the State Sewerage Commission permitted the formation of sewage districts where the consent of the municipalities in the proposed district could be obtained. It was anticipated that the communities of the Passaic Valley would band together for joint action on a trunk sewer. Newark at length asked other towns and cities to join with her in the creation of a sewage board, but the response was not promising.[15]

To move matters off dead center, in April 1901 the Newark Board of Trade arranged a mass meeting of the political, business, and civic leaders of the affected communities to appeal to the governor for the calling of a special legislative session. At the meeting, which was attended by the governor, speakers warned of the health perils and of the likely departure of great manufacturing firms if relief was not forthcoming. The governor was said to be "evidently impressed" and, while the legislature was not called into special session, $8,000 was made available from the governor's emergency fund to the State Sewerage Commission, which was directed to undertake a new and full inquiry into the subject.[16]

The State Sewerage Commission hired William Brown, J.J.R. Croes, and Rudolph Hering, three engineers of national repute, to devise a general system of sewage disposal for the lower Passaic River Valley. The engineers narrowed their choice to two alternative trunk sewer plans: one providing for the discharge of raw sewage at Robbins Reef in upper New York Bay, where strong tidal currents would sweep it out to sea; and the other calling for the disposal of sewage which had undergone primary treatment in Newark Bay. The engineers recommended adoption of the first plan on the grounds that the New York outfall was a final solution and, in the long run, the cheaper remedy.

The legislature approved the work of the State Sewerage Commission and in 1902 passed enabling legislation to permit the construction of a trunk sewer emptying into New York Bay. A separate sewerage district for the Passaic Valley was created and an executive body, the Passaic Valley Sewerage Commissioners, composed of five members appointed from the district by the governor for terms of five years each, was chosen. The district comprised the territory drained by the Passaic River and its tributaries, from the Great Falls at Paterson to Newark Bay, containing about eighty square miles. In 1900 its population was almost 500,000. The route of the proposed intercepting sewer was from the Great Falls along the western bank of the Passaic River to a point in the city of Newark, where it was to leave the river and pass southeasterly through the city, across the Newark salt meadows, continuing under Newark Bay in pipes, across the Bayonne peninsula, and from there to its terminus at Robbins Reef in upper New York Bay, a little more than two miles from the New Jersey shore. The Passaic Valley Sewerage Commission was authorized to finance the project by issuing bonds funded through taxes levied by the commission on property in the district.[17]

At this juncture the city of Paterson, one of the worst despoilers of the river, commenced action to prevent the commission from executing its mandate. Because of its location on the Great Falls, Paterson escaped the worst effects of the river's pollution. The city had been the defendant in several suits—nearly all unsuccessful—for recovery of losses resulting from its discharge of sewage and industrial wastes. Paterson had consistently resisted efforts to force its participation in a trunk sewer scheme. The city argued that it could operate a sewage treatment plant for less than it would cost to dispose of its wastes through a trunk sewer. After first winning a one-year delay in the work, Paterson caused a writ of certiorari to be taken challenging the commission's authority. On appeal to the Court of Errors and Appeals, Paterson in 1905 won its case, the court holding that it was unconstitutional for the legislature to delegate taxation powers to a nonelective body. The part of the statute not relating to taxation was allowed to stand but, shorn of its financial powers, the commission was powerless to undertake any further ventures.[18]

Paterson's victory proved short-lived. The Passaic River's condition was so foul and the dangers to health and property were so manifest as to permit of no further delay in the waterway's purification. To get around the constitutional roadblock raised by the Court of Errors and Appeals, the state in 1907 enacted legislation enabling any or all of the twenty municipalities within the sewerage district to enter into a joint contract with each other and with the Passaic Valley Sewerage Commission for the construction of a trunk sewer. To compel the communities that polluted the river to act on the plan with haste, the statute prohibited the discharge of untreated sewage into the Passaic River or its tributaries after December 12, 1912. The cost of constructing the sewer system was to be paid for by the participating municipalities in direct proportion to their ratables for the year 1907; maintenance and operation expenses were to be borne annually on the basis of use.[19]

Newark and Paterson responded to the state's prodding for the construction of an intercepting sewer along the Passaic River in diametrically opposed ways. Though the cost formula stipulated in the law saddled Newark with more than 50 percent of the building costs, estimated at from $12.25 million to $13.25 million, the city vigorously promoted the trunk sewer plan and helped finance some of the preliminary survey work. Hence Newark was prepared to pay as much for this one sewer as it had spent on all its other sewers. Paterson, on the other hand, had steadfastly opposed the project from its inception. At the time of the Court of Errors and Appeals' decision against the trunk sewer, the *Paterson Evening News* and *The* [Paterson] *Morning Call* had commented that the sewer would have bankrupted the city. The *News* had stated that, with few exceptions, the city was united against the trunk sewer.[20]

Following the passage of the Passaic Valley Sewerage Commission bill in 1907, Paterson engaged "the highest engineering talent" in the hope of finding some other method of satisfying the state's decree. The question was reviewed by eminent engineers and by special committees of Paterson officials and business leaders, who concluded that if raw sewage could be emptied into New York Bay and if the cost estimates of the engineers of the Passaic Valley Sewerage Commission were accurate, a trunk sewer would offer the best expedient. Paterson's pro rata share of the construction costs was 16.5 percent, which amounted to slightly over $2 million (based on a cost estimate of $12.25 million). The mayor feared the actual cost would be much higher, as had been the experience of other cities with major public works projects. For several years Paterson tried to get the Passaic Valley Sewerage Commissioners to secure an estimate on the cost of the sewer from outside engineers or contractors. Failing in this, Paterson, along with other Passaic Valley communities, conducted an extensive study of municipal sewage treatment in the hope of finding an alternative to the trunk sewer plan.[21]

In the meantime the suits brought by riparian owners for recovery of damages arising out of Paterson's pollution of the Passaic River again came up. By 1910 Paterson had paid out $30,000 in damage claims. The awards made to successful plaintiffs, the expense of litigation, and newspaper stories of pending suits were hurting the city's credit rating. The Court of Chancery in an earlier decision had given Paterson until March 26, 1911, to end its pollution of the river. The Passaic Valley Sewerage Commission increased the pressure by declaring a deadline of July 15, 1911, for Paterson to join in the trunk sewer venture.

As the deadline set by the Passaic Valley Sewerage Commissioners approached, Paterson found itself confronted with the prospects of punitive legal action and with its options expired. Since Paterson had proposed no other means of sewage disposal, the Vice Chancellor of the Court of Chancery ordered the city to enter into the trunk sewer plan. Moreover, he threatened to prosecute pending damage suits and hinted at contempt of court proceedings if a contract was not signed. Support for the trunk sewer project was contained in a report by engineer Charles R. Parmlee in July of 1911 for the Paterson Board of Finance. Parmlee had secured a bid for the proposed sewer work from one of the largest contracting firms in the nation. He projected a cost of $13.25 million, which was in line with the $12.25 million estimate of the Passaic Valley Sewerage Commission, the difference in the two appraisals being attributed to a rise in labor costs from the time when the commission had made its estimate. Nevertheless, two days before the commission's deadline, Mayor Andrew F. McBride publicly proclaimed that he would not sign the contract unless the commission gave him definite assurances of the sewer's costs. The commission held its ground, and on July 14 McBride capitulated.[22]

Paterson newspapers did not try to hide their dismay over the city's forced participation in the trunk sewer plan. *The Morning Call* remarked bitterly that "Paterson has been literally clubbed and steam rollered into the scheme, willy, nilly." In opposing the project the *Call* claimed to represent nine-tenths of the people of Paterson. The editors of both *The Morning Call* and the *Paterson Evening News* commented that the work could drag on for years and the cost exceed the original estimate by millions of dollars. The *News*'s editor pointed to engineering studies that calculated an ultimate cost of $20 million. He also noted the enormous expense of tunneling beneath Newark Bay and the Bayonne peninsula should it become necessary to build a sewage treatment plant on the Newark salt meadows to satisfy the objections to the project that had been raised by the United States Government.[23] The mayor in his annual report commented that the sewer could increase Paterson's bonded indebtedness by as much as 50 percent. However, he put the best face on the matter by observing that the resolution of the dispute opened the way for an extension of sewerage in the West Paterson and Totowa sections of town, neither of which had "had the increase in population to which they are entitled, because of lack of proper sewage facilities."[24] The Passaic Valley Sewerage Commission, of course, was jubilant. The signing of Paterson brought the number of municipalities which had joined in the project to fifteen, including all of those adjacent to the river.

New difficulties arose as the plan entered final preparations. Residents of the great metropolis across the Hudson River had been watching the progress made on the trunk sewer with apprehension. The decision reached by the State Sewerage Commission in 1902 to put the outlet of the sewer in New York Bay had prompted the creation of the New York Bay Pollution Commission. After studying the question from 1903 to 1906, this commission had recommended that New York State seek an injunction against the sewer. It had been aided in its investigation by business and historic conservation groups, including the Merchants' Association of New York, the New York Chamber of Commerce, the New York Produce Exchange, the Maritime Exchange, and the American Scenic and Historic Preservation Society.[25]

The state of New York followed up the report of the New York Bay Pollution Commission by establishing the Metropolitan Sewerage Commission of New York and by bringing suit in the United States Supreme Court against the Passaic Valley Sewerage Commission and the state of New Jersey. The United States Government then requested and obtained permission to intervene in the suit and become a co-plaintiff. United States government authorities feared that the discharge of sewage into New York Bay would choke the Narrows, hindering navigation at the big port. They were also concerned about the sewage from the flume damaging United States property in the harbor and endangering the public health. To overcome the objections of the United States Government, the defendants in 1911 agreed to remove solid particles and grit from the sewage through screening and sedimentation. The Passaic Valley Sewerage Commissioners also consented to secure an absence in New York Bay of visible suspended particles, of deposits objectionable to the Secretary of War, and of odors due to the putrefaction of organic matter contained in the Passaic Valley sewage thus discharged; they further agreed that there would be no injury to federal property or public health, no public or private nuisance, and no reduction in the dissolved oxygen content of the waters of New York Bay that would interfere with major fish life as a result of the commission's operations.[26]

New York State, however, at the behest of New York City, pressed ahead with the suit. The Metropolitan Sewerage Commission of New York argued that the degree of purification agreed to by the Passaic Valley Sewerage Commissioners was insufficient because it encompassed only the removal of solid particles and made no reference to dissolved organic matter. This imperfect purification, the commission protested, invited putrefaction and would lead to a repulsive stench which, when the wind was blowing in a northeasterly direction, would waft over the densely crowded downtown section of New York City. Furthermore, the commission stated that the plan to disperse the Passaic Valley sewage through 150 widely scattered outlets over a 3½ acre area 40 feet beneath the surface of the sea was experimental and hence risky. Finally, the commission complained that the agreement entered into between the United States Government and the Passaic Valley Sewerage Commissioners should be enforced by the City or State of New York or an interstate commission, and not by the Secretary of War, who had no responsibility of a sanitary nature toward the people of New York. The United States Supreme Court disagreed, and in 1916 ruled against the plaintiff, leaving the way open for the completion of the trunk sewer.[27]

Even with this final obstacle to the construction of the Passaic Valley Trunk Sewer removed, the project continued to cause anguish for Newark and Paterson. Work on the sewer had begun in 1912 but was held up by the United States Supreme Court case, and then again by the entry of the United States into World War I. The delays in the project forced the State of New Jersey to keep postponing the date for prohibiting the discharge of untreated sewage into the Passaic River. The *Newark Evening News* reported on October 31, 1917, that the Passaic River "still smells to heaven" and its acid fumes were peeling the paint from buildings all along the waterway from Paterson to Newark Bay.

The apprehensions Paterson had about the ultimate cost of the sewer proved well founded. The original trunk sewer proposal, envisioning the discharge of sewage into New York Bay by a gravity flow, could not be carried out because of the United States Government stipulation that the sewage be treated. Instead, it forced the building of a pumping station on the Newark salt meadows which, in turn, had to be connected with the dispersion system in New York Bay. The connection involved tunneling under conditions which could not be accurately determined in advance, and, when water was discovered in the strata underlying Newark Bay, the construction of a five-mile outfall pressure tunnel became necessary. These complications increased the cost of the sewer and still further delayed its completion. An even more important factor in the sewer's spiraling cost was the inflation caused by World War I. Twice the Passaic Valley Sewerage Commissioners had to appeal to the participating municipalities for additional appropriations. The final cost of the trunk sewer, as Paterson had foreseen, was $21 million. Meanwhile the threat to Newark manufacturers posed by the stench and fumes of the river led Newark to appeal to the Passaic Valley Sewerage Commissioners for relief. A committee of Newark engineers in 1920 proposed to dispose of sewage effluent from the treatment plant into the upper waters of Newark Bay for a period not exceeding five years while work on the trunk sewer continued. The commissioners rejected the plea and the sewer was completed in 1924, twelve years after the work had first started.[28]

The Passaic Valley Trunk Sewer drains a district in northern New Jersey about eighty square miles in area, extending from Paterson in the north to Newark in the south, and from the Orange Mountains in the west to the watershed divide between the Passaic and Hackensack valleys in the east. At the time of its opening in 1924 it served twenty-two municipalities whose population in 1932 exceeded one million.[29] The pumping station on the meadows was designed to handle 100 million gallons a day with space provided for the installation of new machinery which would increase its capacity substantially beyond that. J. Ralph Van Duyne, the chief engineer of the Passaic Valley Sewerage Commissioners, in 1932 reported a significant increase in the oxygen content of the water, indicating that pollution had been diminished, but the river never regained its earlier fame and beauty.[30] The *American City Magazine* in its October 1924 issue celebrated the completion of the sewer and recounted the vicissitudes through which it had passed. It noted prophetically that though the sewer's capacity had been expanded beyond the limits planned in 1912, when it was projected that the sewer would be adequate until 1940, "some years hence the municipalities along the Passaic will again be forced to discuss an extension of the sewerage works."[31]

NOTES

1. *Newark Evening News*, May 23, 1884; Hugh Holmes, *Reminiscences of 75 Years of Belleville, Franklin, and Newark* (2d ed., n.p., 1895 or 1896), pp. 53-54.

2. *Newark Athletic Club News* (Feb. 1921), pp. 19-20; *Sunday Call*, Feb. 19, 1933; *Newark Evening News*, April 17, 1949, April 22, 1956; *Newark Star-Ledger*, July 20, 1946.

3. Frank John Urquhart, *A History of the City of Newark, New Jersey* (3 vols.; New York: The Lewis Historical Publishing Co., 1913), II, 670-2.

4. *Newark Star-Ledger*, July 20, 1946.

5. N.J., *Report of the Passaic Valley Sewerage Commission, 1897*, pp. 1-14.

6. Daniel Jacobson, "The Pollution Problem of the Passaic River," *Proceedings of the New Jersey Historical Society*, LIV (July 1958), 186-98.

7. N.J., *Annual Report of the State Sewerage Commission, 1905*, p. 8 (hereinafter referred to as *ARSSC*); N.J., State Water Supply Commission, *Annual Report, 1908*, p. 6.

8. *Newark Evening News*, May 23, 1884; Anon., *History of Passaic Valley District Sewerage and Drainage Commission* (n.p., n.d.); Urquhart, *Newark*, II, 672; *Newark Star-Ledger*, July 20, 1946.

9. *Sunday Call*, May 18, 1890.

10. *Newark Evening News*, April 22, 1956.

11. *ARNJBH, 1895*, pp. 8-25.

12. *Annual Report of the Board of Trade, 1897*, p. 15. Representing Newark on the commission were H.C.H. Herold, the president of the board of health, and William T. Hunt, the editor of the *Sunday Call*.

13. *ARSSC, 1905*, pp. 5-6; N.J., *Senate Journal* (1897), *Governor's Message with Reference to Pollution of the Passaic River and a General System of Sewerage Disposal for the Valley of the Passaic*, pp. 356-7; *Communication from Passaic Valley Sewerage Commissioners to Honorable Thomas L. Raymond . . . Reviewing Report of Committee of Engineers Concerning Passaic Valley Sewer Project* (1920), pp. 24-30, 51 (herein-

PLATE III

PASSAIC VALLEY SEWERAGE SYSTEM

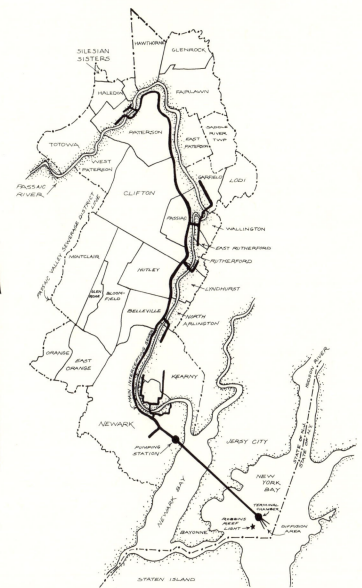

SOURCE: New Jersey, Report of the Passaic Valley Sewerage Commissioners,
1924-1949 (n.p.:_____,n.d.).

after referred to as *Communication from Passaic Valley Sewerage Commissioners to Honorable Thomas L. Raymond); Newark Evening News,* December 24, 1901.

14. William Edgar Sackett, *Modern Battles of Trenton: Being a History of New Jersey Politics and Legislation from the Year 1868 to the Year 1894* (2 vols.; Trenton, N.J.: John L. Murphy, Printer, 1895), II, 141; *Newark Evening News,* Feb. 3, 1898, April 21, 1901. Newark Board of Trade, *Yearbook, 1899,* p. 13.

15. *ARSSC, 1905,* pp. 6-7; *Sunday Call,* March 26, 1899, Nov. 4, Dec. 16, 1900. One sewer, the Joint Outlet or Suburban Joint Sewer, was built under the law. It serviced western Newark and five neighboring municipalities in Union and Essex counties, and discharged its wastes into the waters of Arthur Kill; *ARSSC,* 1902, pp. 8-9.

16. *Newark Evening News,* April 18, 1901; *ARSSC, 1905,* pp. 9-10.

17. *ARSSC, 1905,* pp. 7-8; *Communication from Passaic Valley Sewerage Commissioners to Honorable Thomas L. Raymond,* pp. 51-53; *State of New York v. State of New Jersey and Passaic Valley Sewerage Commissioners,* 4 U.S. 3069-70 (1916).

18. *ARSSC, 1905,* p. 8; *Sunday Call,* March 5, 12, 1901; *Paterson Evening News,* March 7, 1905; *The* [Paterson] *Morning Call,* March 7, 1905.

19. *State of New York v. New Jersey and Passaic Valley Sewerage Commissioners,* 1 U.S. 15-22 (1916).

20. Taylor, *Passaic Valley Sewerage Commission,* pp. 5-6; *Sunday Call,* April 26, 1908; *Paterson Evening News,* March 7, 1905; *The* [Paterson] *Morning Call,* March 7, 1905.

21. *Annual Report of the City Officers of the City of Paterson, New Jersey, 1910, Mayor's Message,* pp. 51-53 (hereinafter referred to as *Paterson Annual Reports,* year); *Paterson Evening News,* July 13-14, 1911; *The* [Paterson] *Morning Call,* July 14, 1911.

22. *Paterson Annual Reports, 1910, Mayor's Message,* pp. 51-53, *1911,* pp. 32-34; *Paterson Evening News,* July 13-14, 1911; *The* [Paterson] *Morning Call,* July 14, 1911.

23. *The* [Paterson] *Morning Call,* July 13-14, 1911; *Paterson Evening News,* July 14, 1911.

24. *Paterson Annual Reports, 1911, Mayor's Message,* p. 33.

25. Metropolitan Sewerage Commission of New York, *Report on the Discharge of Sewage from the Proposed Passaic Valley Sewer of New Jersey, May 23, 1910,* pp. 1-2 (hereinafter referred to as Metropolitan Sewerage Commission of New York, *Report on Passaic Valley Sewer Discharge).*

26. Ibid., p. 6; *State of New York v. State of New Jersey and Passaic Valley Sewerage Commissioners,* 1 U.S. 26-27, 108-9, 5 U.S. 4006-8 (1916).

27. Metropolitan Sewerage Commission of New York, *Report on Passaic Valley Sewer Discharge*, pp. 2-6; "Passaic Valley Trunk Sewer Completed," *The American City Magazine* (Oct. 1924), p. 318; *State of New York v. State of New Jersey and Passaic Valley Sewerage Commissioners*, 1 U.S. 27-29 (1916).

28. *Communication from Passaic Valley Sewerage Commissioners to Honorable Thomas L. Raymond*, pp. 5-10, 44-49; N.J., *Report of the Passaic Valley Sewerage Commissioners, 1929-1949* (n.p., n.d.), pp. 5-7.

29. The original municipalities participating in the trunk sewer plan were: Newark, Paterson, Passaic, Harrison, Kearny, Belleville, Clifton, Nutley, East Newark, Garfield, Lyndhurst, Rutherford, East Rutherford, Wallington, and North Arlington. Municipalities which joined later included: Orange, East Orange, Montclair, Prospect Park, Haledon, Glen Ridge, and Bloomfield.

30. J. Ralph Van Duyne, "Eight Years' Operation of Passaic Valley Sewer," *Engineering News-Record* (Oct. 13, 1932), p. 28.

31. "Passaic Valley Trunk Sewer Completed," *The American City Magazine* (Oct. 1924), p. 317.

6

Mosquito Extermination

Newark's first settlers built their homes on high ground away from the tidal marshes which surrounded them on two sides. To the south lay the Great Salt Meadow, a tidal swampland embracing about one-third of present-day Newark and part of northern Elizabeth. Several streams, two of which were navigable, meandered through the meadows amidst countless ponds, the bigger ones an acre or more in size. In wet weather the streams swelled and the ponds multiplied, transforming the meadows into an impenetrable watery wasteland. To the east, across the Passaic River, stretched the huge Hackensack meadows, an area of marsh grass, cedar swamps, and cattails, still today only partially reclaimed.

Though Newark's founders avoided the heat and humidity of the meadows, they could not escape the stings of the mosquitoes that bred there. Every spring and summer, great broods of salt marsh mosquitoes arose from the meadows to bring discomfort and illness to the people of Newark.[1]

"Newark was known the civilized world over for its mosquitoes and its cider, for many generations."[2] At night it was impossible to sleep without screens and mosquito net canopies. Often even this protection was insufficient. In the morning the harried victim sought revenge by attaching a can of kerosene to the end of a broom handle and pressing it against the blood-filled mosquitoes resting on the ceiling. It is reported that the insects' presence sometimes forced businesses to close.[3] The torments of the mosquit especially at night, were legion: sleeping children were tortured, outdoor sporting events were canceled, and families were denied the delights of a summer evening on the porch. In the summertime many left Newark for resort areas with the sole purpose of escaping the pest.[4]

The mosquitoes of the Newark area were known for their size and voraciousness. Washington Irving described Newark as "noted for its fine breed of fat mosquitoes, [which are able to] sting through the thickest

boot."[5] A traveler who had taken the road from New York to Newark
across the Hackensack meadows remarked that "they will continue sucking
your blood, if not disturbed, till they swell to four times their ordinary
size, when they absolutely fall off and burst from their fullness."[6]

The mosquitoes were more than a nuisance, for certain varieties carried
in their bodies the parasites responsible for malaria. Correspondents to the
Essex County Medical Society regularly reported that "intermittent and
remittent fevers prevailed in early spring, and continued through the season
till near winter."[7] The state health commission of 1874 stated that Newark
had at times "suffered greatly,"[8] and "the town appears also to have early
obtained the character abroad of being an uninhabitable place—subject to
fever and agues and 'intermittents,' which is supposed to have retarded its
growth."[9]

Malaria, a disease of the red blood cells, is characterized by paroxysms of
fever and chills occurring at regular intervals measured in days (tertian
malaria; quartan malaria). The sequelae of a bout of malaria are severely
debilitating. Victims of the disease undergo long periods of protracted
illness and have less resistance to other infections. The malady is recurrent
and relapses are frequent.[10] In certain counties of New Jersey it was a fortunate individual who did not suffer every year from repeated attacks of
malaria. The disease wreaked havoc upon newcomers and claimed its
victims principally among the infirm, the aged, and the very young.[11]

Malaria is transmitted through the bite of the female anopheles mosquito. The insect thrives in clear fresh water amidst the sheltering vegetation
found along the banks of streams, ponds, and lakes. Turbulence and salt
water are inimical to most kinds of anopheles mosquitoes.[12]

Though salt marshes do not provide a natural habitat for most species of
anopheles mosquito, the Great Salt Meadows was a vast incubator of
malaria. For one thing, it contained numerous bodies of fresh water; for
another thing, there is considerable overlapping of one species of mosquito
on the territory of another. In addition, the *anopheles quadrimaculatus,*
the principal carrier of malaria in New Jersey, is capable of breeding in
the brackish water of salt marshes and enjoys a somewhat greater range
than that of most species of malarial mosquitoes.[13] That fevers and agues
were more or less endemic in the wards bordering the Newark salt meadows,
wrote Dr. Lott Southard, "none can deny."[14]

Malaria can be treated with quinine, an alkaloid derived from the bark of
certain trees of the genus cinchona, which grow in South America. Use of

quinine arrests the progress of the disease, but the germ remains in the body, and the individual must guard against a recrudescence of the parasitemia. The cinchona bark was brought to Europe from Peru around 1630; quinine, its active ingredient, was isolated in 1820. Misuse of the drug caused a reaction against its prescription, and quinine was regarded as a backup treatment to the usual bloodletting, antimony, and opiates. The administration of quinine in large doses to American soldiers during the Seminole War of the late 1830s and early 1840s established the effectiveness of the drug, and in the second half of the nineteenth century it was consumed in enormous quantities. But though quinine gave relief, it could not break the chain of infection. Consequently, malaria remained rampant wherever the anopheles mosquito flourished.[15]

The nineteenth century witnessed the apex of malaria's destructiveness in the United States. Malaria waited in ambush for the settlers as they moved into the great river valleys of the Midwest. River bottoms, bayous, and other places of stagnant water were especially unhealthful. Malaria and dysentery made invalids of river valley inhabitants, many of whom migrated to the Southwest in the hope of recovering their health. The pale, gaunt, and emaciated appearance of those that remained behind became a national sterotype. New England experienced a resurgence of malaria in the years 1870-1890 with the return of large numbers of Civil War veterans who had contracted the disease.[16] Some of the mid-Atlantic states also fared poorly. The New Jersey State Health Commission of 1874 reported that malaria was the state's principal medical problem. "It, probably more than any other one disease, interferes with our productive labour and is not only like an epidemic but resident, inflicting an annual tax upon the individual resources of our State, and upon the comfort of its citizens."[17] In the South malaria remained endemic until well into the twentieth century. More illness was caused in the United States by malaria than by any other pestilence.

The advance of civilization proved inimical to the disease. Concomitant with urbanization was a decline in the incidence of malaria. Municipal improvements such as sewer construction, street paving, and the draining of small swampy patches eliminated local breeding areas. By 1900 mosquito breeding grounds had been pushed beyond the range of most American cities.[18] In the rural reaches of the Upper Mississippi Valley the arrest of new inward migrations, cultivation of the land, screening, better housing, and the raising of dairy cattle brought about a decline in malaria which antedated by decades organized drainage enterprises.[19]

It was long observed that malaria was common near mill sites and swamps and did not occur when the weather turned cold. Miasma, however, and not the mosquito, was held accountable (the word malaria means "bad air"). The role of vectors in transmitting disease was not known until Sir Ronald Ross's work with malaria in India and Walter Reed's experiments with yellow fever in Cuba around the turn of the twentieth century.[20] (A Newark nurse, Clara Maass, acted as a guinea pig in Reed's experiments, whereupon she became ill and died. A Newark hospital is now named in her honor.)[21]

On the basis of their encounters with tidal marshes in Connecticut, Newark's founders were able to find a use for the meadows bordering their new home. Once the marsh grass in the more accessible areas had been burned, salt hay, which was used as bedding and forage for livestock, could be grown. When the lots in the "Town Plot" were divided, each citizen was assigned a section of the Newark salt meadows.

The decline of farming in the Newark area in the nineteenth century ended the usefulness of the Great Salt Meadows. The Hackensack meadows suffered a similar fate. Diversion of the upstream waters of the Hackensack River led to increased salt water intrusion. The burning of the meadows, the overcutting of the good stands of timber, and the alterations in the contour of the land brought about by the construction of railroad enbankments and by ditching and diking destroyed the region's economic value. Cattails took over most of the Hackensack meadows north of Kearny. This, at least, had the beneficial consequence of crowding out the mosquito. Farmers continued to dike and partially reclaim small parcels, and pig farms thrived in Secaucus, but primarily the meadows provided sites for transportation depots and garbage dumps. Unwanted, untouched, and uninhabited, the Hackensack and Newark meadows became wastelands.[22]

The first comprehensive plan for reclaiming the meadows was prepared by a committee appointed by the common council in 1859. The committee envisioned the region as a center for truck farming. A state legislative commission was appointed to execute the work, and about $2,000 was spent on diking and construction of tide gates.[23]

In the years immediately following the Civil War, malaria flared up in Newark. The outbreak was attributed to faulty diking, which had interfered with the natural drainage of the meadows. This, it was believed, had aggravated the miasma in the area, causing the increased sickness. Faulty diking was partially responsible for the epidemic, but not for the reason given. Diking operations had brought about the formation of a great number of stagnant ponds on the meadows and had prevented the salt water that normally came in with the tide from inundating fresh water pools. The mosquitoes that bred in these pools had fed on returning soldiers with malaria, causing the epidemic. Because of the presence of malaria, coupled with high prices and a scarcity of labor, work on the reclamation of the meadows was halted in 1868. A short time thereafter work was resumed briefly and then about 1880 was abandoned once more.[24]

In 1866 a company with assets of $11 million was incorporated by the New Jersey State Legislature to construct a ship canal from New York Bay to downtown Newark via the Bayonne peninsula and the Newark salt meadows. The project attracted considerable attention and for a number of years the proposed canal was shown on city directory maps. A small amount of excavation was done, but other than that nothing came of the scheme.[25] Another million-dollar corporation was formed in 1870 to reclaim the meadows, whose accomplishments were even less tangible than those of the ship canal company. In 1872 the common council committee on sewers and drainage was instructed to report on a plan for salvaging the meadows. The committee recommended that the meadows be filled to a height of from five to eight feet above high water with material dredged from Newark Bay. Not for nearly forty years would the committee's plan be realized.[26]

In the 1880s the board of trade became interested in the meadows question. Faced with rising land costs, the likelihood of higher taxes, and the need to acquire new industrial sites, Newark business leaders looked to the development of the meadows for relief. The time also seemed propitious for Newark to challenge the commercial preeminence of New York, which had allowed its port to deteriorate. Mechanization of cargo handling was rapidly making New York's piers obsolete. Adequate terminal and freight facilities were lacking, costs were high, the harbor was congested, and expensive delays attended the movement of goods. Newark, with its vast undeveloped meadows, possessed a great potential competitive advantage over New York. If an oceangoing port was established on Newark Bay and if the meadows were reclaimed, then the railroads that passed through the area on their way to New York could be diverted to terminal-docking facilities on the meadows, and a large part of the business of transshipping goods would fall Newark's way.[27]

In 1885 the board of trade published a pamphlet outlining its plan for reclamation of the meadows. The proposal won the support of the common council, but was vetoed by the mayor because of fear that malaria and other diseases would result from the decomposition of the vegetable matter left exposed to the sun while construction was under way. In addition, the mayor was wary of the scheme's cost and feasibility.[28]

About 1890 an effort was made by the city to untangle the web of conflicting land ownership titles that had been forming since the time of the original distribution of lots in the seventeenth century. A study was made of all extant ownership deeds and the area was surveyed and mapped. "With taxes to pay, the owners became aware that these supposedly worthless lands had some value and certain far seeing citizens began to buy up and consolidate small tracts into large holdings."[29] In 1897 the State Geological Survey endorsed a plan embracing the use of dikes and pumps to drain the meadows.[30]

In 1899 the board of trade announced it would award a prize of $1,000 for the best plan submitted on the problem. The board of works got behind the drive for meadow reclamation, and in a referendum held in 1907 the city voters approved a $1 million municipal appropriation to make it a reality.[31]

Along with Newark, many other areas of New Jersey were infested with mosquitoes. The greater part of the state consists of a low-lying coastal plain. Bordering the state's offshore waters, comprising Newark Bay, Raritan Bay, the Atlantic Ocean, and Delaware Bay, are extensive coastal salt marshes. Inland there are vast tidal marshes along the Hackensack River and many upland breeding areas in Morris and Burlington counties.[32] "Early in the twentieth century New Jersey earned for itself the sobriquet of the 'Mosquito State,' and outsiders spoke of the 'Jersey Mosquito' as if it were an especially large and voracious species *sui generis.* "[33]

Before 1900 few New Jerseyites paid much attention to the mosquito. The mosquito was viewed as an affliction of nature, something to be made light of and endured as one did hay fever or poison ivy. No one thought seriously about eliminating the mosquito, causing the *Sunday Call* to comment that

> the custom has been to laugh at the mosquito pest, as sea sickness is ridiculed, but when the mosquito causes financial ruin to hotel keepers, prevents the sale of land, brings nervous trouble upon victims, prevents needed rest, and compels large expenditures by those who find it necessary to get relief; when we find that the whole State of

New Jersey gets a bad name from the pest, and when men of science tell us that many forms of malarial troubles are probably due to the bites, the mosquito ceases to be a laughing matter.[34]

Leading the fight against the mosquito in New Jersey was Dr. John B. Smith, the State Entomologist at the New Jersey Agricultural Experiment Station. In 1901 Smith began his campaign by sending inquiries to local health officials on the incidence of malaria and the extent of the mosquito problem in their communities. With this knowledge and with information acquired from a projected study of New Jersey mosquitoes, Smith envisioned a statewide scientifically directed program of mosquito extermination. At the time the idea of mosquito eradication seemed farfetched, and when in 1902 Smith appealed to the legislature for funds, his proposal was greeted with laughter.

The governor had more faith in the plan and provided money for a demonstration project. The response to the project, which Smith took around the state, was enthusiastic, and in the following year the legislature reversed itself. Subsequently, there appeared in 1905 Smith's epic "Report of the New Jersey State Agricultural Experiment Station upon the Mosquitoes Occurring Within the State, Their Habits, Life History, etc." In this work Smith described the characteristics and habits of every mosquito species found in New Jersey along with the measures necessary for their control. The report revealed that more than half of the state's land surface, containing upward of three-quarters of its population, was overrun with mosquitoes.[35]

A grant-in-aid program was begun in which the state agreed to assume one-fourth of the costs of mosquito extermination. Newark, Elizabeth, and other communities bordering the Newark salt meadows quickly responded to the state's offer and from 35,000 to 40,000 feet of ditches were dug in the worst places.[36] In addition, the Newark Board of Health spent about $1,000 annually during the years 1904-1910 distributing crude oil and oiling catch basins. In 1911 the board assigned a full-time inspector to mosquito and fly control.[37]

At the behest of the Newark Board of Health, in the summer of 1903 delegates from nineteen boards of health in Essex and Hudson counties established a "Conference Committee on Mosquito Extermination." In 1904 the committee secured the passage of a bill empowering local boards of health to abate mosquito breeding nuisances. In 1910 the name of the association was changed to the North Jersey Mosquito Extermination

League. The League acted as both a lobby and a clearinghouse for information. In 1912 its functions were assumed by county mosquito extermination commissions, and the league was disbanded.[38]

Financing mosquito extermination elsewhere throughout the state
proved to be a snare. Few communities availed themselves of the state
grant-in-aid program. In 1905 $350,000 was made available to the Agri-
cultural Experiment Station for use as seed money, but again there were
few takers.[39]

> The Agricultural Experiment Station did manage though, with the
> 'noble' participation of Newark, Jersey City and Elizabeth, all of
> whom footed nearly all of the bills themselves, to do considerable
> work in the marsh areas. Thousands of acres of meadowland were
> treated and millions of feet of drainage ditches were dug. New Jersey
> was said to stand 'first in mosquito warfare' among the states in
> 1911.[40]

Even in the Newark area, however, the state was only partially successful in eliminating the mosquito nuisance. Though the salt water mosquito
was almost eradicated from the Newark-Elizabeth meadows area, wrigglers
hatched in the Hackensack meadows near Kearny continued to plague
the city. Municipalities were shackled in fighting the mosquito by their
inability to destroy mosquito breeding grounds that lay outside their
corporate limits. In 1908 the Newark Board of Health temporarily abandoned
its mosquito work when it found it could provide only transient relief from
the pest. Insects are not respecters of political boundaries. If mosquito
extermination was to be effective, then it would have to be made mandatory
in every county.[41]

In 1912 the New Jesey State Legislature passed legislation requiring
the creation of county mosquito extermination commissions. The director
of the Agricultural Experiment Station was made the coordinator of the
program and was granted the authority to pass on the plans submitted
by the commissions and on the sums appropriated for their completion.[42]

In 1912 the Essex County Mosquito Extermination Commission became
one of the first commissions to begin operation under the law. To enable
the commission to get started immediately, money was borrowed in the
spring of 1912 in anticipation of taxes due in December of that year. The
New Jersey Board of Health exhibited the commission's accomplishments
for the first year as a model for other commissions to emulate.[43]

The commission's work had two phases: 1) elimination of the salt

marsh mosquito; and 2) extermination of the fresh water mosquito. In
the summer of 1912 a house-to-house inspection was made in Newark. The
target of the drive was the common house mosquito, *Culex Pipiens,* a fresh
water mosquito that breeds in stagnant pools near human habitation. Manure
pits, privy vaults, wells, cisterns, sewer and catch basins, rain barrels, watering
troughs, roof gutters, flooded basements, rain pools, swampy patches, and
the overgrown edges of streams are its most common breeding grounds.
During the winter of 1912-1913 over ten thousand mosquito marshes were
drained, filled in, oiled, or otherwise made harmless. The results obtained
were said to surpass all expectations. Corroborating the commission's
boasts, there was a sharp decline in the sale of mosquito canopies and oil
of citronella.[44] By the end of 1915 the fresh water mosquito was vanquished

Special attention was paid to the Newark salt meadows. During the
winter of 1912-1913 the area was surveyed and laid out in ten-acre plots.
Ditches were dug to carry off water from poorly drained sections of the
meadows and to supplement inadequate natural outlet streams. Standing
ditch water was stocked with predatory fish life or was oiled. Over
500,000 feet of new ditches were built which, when added to the footage
constructed prior to 1912, brought the total to over 1 million feet.[46]

Snags developed, however, in the commission's work on the meadows.
Tidal action filled the ditches with large amounts of residue, necessitating
frequent dredging. During prolonged periods of adverse weather the
drainage system broke down. In July 1913 two weeks of heavy rains, high
tides, and unfavorable winds made the meadows too water-laden for
travel. By the time men were able to get in to apply oil to the new breeding
areas, it was too late, for the mosquitoes had already hatched.

The 1913 debacle forced a change in the project's modus operandi.
It was decided to "Hollandize" the salt meadows, i.e., to free the area of
tide and storm water through the use of dikes and tide gates. Dikes were
built around the margin of the salt marsh and automatic tide gates were
constructed at outlet streams. Even then the drainage was inadequate.
Torrential downpours in August of the following year caused a break in
the dikes and destroyed a tide gate, flooding part of the meadows. The
problem was finally solved by using the Newark sewage pumping station
on the meadows to aid in removing excess water.[47]

In 1914, with the help of the state and federal governments, work was
started on the construction of a deep water channel from the meadows out
to Newark Bay. Newark was destined to become a great rail-to-ship terminal.
To make way for the docking facilities, warehouses, and factories that were

contemplated, the meadows adjacent to the channel had to be reclaimed and developed.[48] World War I lent an air of urgency to the undertaking. Land was needed for war factories, and a shipyard was planned for Port Newark.[49] Reclamation of the salt meadows proceeded "beyond the wildest anticipation of those interested in meadows development."[50] By 1918 the salt marshes of Essex County were 96 percent drained.[51]

Meanwhile, in other areas of the county mosquito extermination was making significant progress.[52] For a period Essex County continued to suffer from mosquitoes hatched in Bergen and Hudson counties.[53] Nevertheless, in 1924 the Essex County Mosquito Extermination Commission could report that "at an annual cost rate of less than 11½ cents per capita, the larger population centers of Essex County had been freed of the mosquito nuisance which only ten years ago [had] made living conditions during the summer months all but intolerable."[54]

By 1924 Newark's only permanent mosquito breeding areas were garbage dumps, sewer catch basins, and the like, which because of their utility could not be eliminated—and these were carefully watched. Henceforth the problem of mosquito control in Newark would be largely one of maintenance and repair.[55]

The benefits resulting from mosquito extermination and meadows reclamation were substantial. Malaria practically disappeared from the mortality tables of Newark,[56] and property values in areas rid of mosquitoes rose sharply. The benefits in northern New Jersey to be realized by mosquito extermination were estimated at $1 billion.[57] Construction of a great ocean port was made possible; subsequently, an airport was built on the meadows. But because of the watery subsoil, the meadows could not be used extensively for industrial sites. Except for some warehousing and light industry, the meadows remain much the same as they were at the time of the airport's completion.[58]

The mosquito situation improved throughout all of New Jersey and remained under control until the mid-1950s when, through neglect and natural forces, the state again became infested with large broods of mosquitoes. The outbreak of eastern encephalitis at this time and the occurrence of malaria among Vietnam veterans served notice of the need for a constant vigil.

NOTES

1. *Sunday Call,* Sept. 4, 1887; *Newark Evening News,* January 29, 1950; *ARNJBH, 1877,* p. 135; Thomas J. Headlee, *The Mosquitoes of New*

Jersey and their Control (New Brunswick, N.J.: Rutgers University Press, 1945), pp. 3-6, 261; Kemble Widmer, *The Geology and Geography of New Jersey*, Vol. XIX of *The New Jersey Historical Series*, eds. Richard M. Huber and Wheaton J. Lane (Princeton, N.J.: D. Van Nostrand Co., Inc., 1964), p. 82.

2. Frank John Urquhart, *A History of the City of Newark, New Jersey* (3 vols.; New York: The Lewis Historical Publishing Co., 1913), I, 38

3. David L. Cowen, *Medicine and Health in New Jersey: A History*, Vol. XVI of The New Jersey Historical Series, eds. Richard M. Huber and Wheaton J. Lane (Princeton, N.J.: D. Van Nostrand Co., Inc., 1964), p. 166

4. *Sunday Call*, January 21, 1906; Essex County, *Annual Report of the Mosquito Extermination Commission, 1932*, pp. 3-4 (hereinafter referred to as *ARECMEC*).

5. Cited in John T. Cunningham, *Newark* (Newark: The New Jersey Historical Society, 1966), p. 94.

6. New Jersey Mosquito Extermination Association, *Proceedings of the Annual Meeting, 1916*, p. 85 (hereinafter referred to as *NJMEA Proceedings*).

7. Anon., "The Climatology and Diseases of Essex County," *Trans. MSNJ, 1887*, pp. 114-38; Joseph A. Vasselli, "A Pestilence Census-Taker in New Jersey," *Bulletin of the History of Medicine*, XXV (1951), 360.

8. New Jersey, *Legislative Documents* (1875), Document No. 24, *Report of the Health Commission for the Year 1874*, p. 19 (hereinafter referred to as *Report of the Health Commission . . . 1874*).

9. *NJMEA Proceedings, 1916*, p. 86. See also Clark, "History of the 'Cholera' Epidemic as it Appeared in the City of Newark, N.J., from June to October, 1849," *New York Journal of Medicine*, N.S., Vol. IV (1850), 211.

10. Frederick B. Bang, "Malaria," Kenneth F. Maxcy and Milton J. Rosenau, *Preventive Medicine and Public Health*, ed. Philip E. Sartwell (9th ed., rev. and enl.; New York: Appleton-Century-Crofts, 1965), pp. 332-3; Charles Wilcocks, *Medical Advance, Public Health, and Social Evolution* (Oxford: Pergamon Press, 1965), pp. 162-5.

11. *ARNJBH, 1877*, pp. 122-3.

12. Wilcocks, *Public Health and Social Evolution*, pp. 162-5.

13. Headlee, *The Mosquitoes of New Jersey*, pp. 8, 92, 102; John B. Smith, *Report of the New Jersey State Agricultural Experimental Station upon the Mosquitoes Occurring within the State, their Habits, Life History*, etc. (Trenton, N.J.: MacCrellish and Quigley, State Printers, 1904), p. 369.

14. *Trans. MSNJ, 1871*, p. 278. See also *Newark Annual Reports, 1880*, *Board of Health*, p. 428; *Sunday Call*, August 20, 1893.

15. John Duffy, *Epidemics in Colonial America* (Baton Rouge, La.: Louisiana State University Press, 1953), p. 243; Bang, "Malaria," p. 334; Erwin H. Ackerknecht, *Malaria in the Upper Mississippi Valley, 1760-1900. Supplements to the Bulletin of the History of Medicine*, No. 4 (Baltimore: The Johns Hopkins Press, 1945), pp. 99-103.

16. Billy M. Jones, *Health Seekers in the Southwest, 1879-1900* (Norman, Oklahoma: University of Oklahoma Press, 1967), pp. 3-22; Ackerknecht, *Malaria*, pp. 129-30.

17. *Report of the Health Commission . . . 1874*, p. 18.

18. Vasselli, "A Pestilence Census-Taker," pp. 363-5; *Trans. MSNJ, 1859*, p. 38; Ackerknecht, *Malaria*, pp. 54-61.

19. Ackerknecht, *Malaria*, pp. 129-30.

20. Cowen, *Medicine and Health in New Jersey*, p. 166.

21. *Newark Evening News*, Jan. 29, 1950; Cunningham, *Newark*, pp. 20, 31; *Sunday Call*, Sept. 4, 1887.

22. *Newark Evening News*, January 29, 1950; Smith, *Report of the New Jersey State Agricultural Experimental Station*, pp. 384-5; Charles C. Morrison, Jr., "The Hackensack Meadows," *Newark, Commerce: Newark Association of Commerce and Industry, Newark, N.J.*, VII, No. 5 (November 1962), pp. 21, 38; *Sunday Call*, September 4, 1887.

23. Edward S. Rankin, *The Running Brooks and Other Sketches of Early Newark* (Somerville, N.J.: The Unionist-Gazette, 1930), pp. 80-81.

24. *Trans. MSNJ, 1869*, pp. 84, 145-6; Rankin, *Sketches of Early Newark*, p. 82; *Newark Annual Reports, 1880, Board of Health*, p. 428.

25. Rankin, *Sketches of Early Newark*, pp. 82-83.

26. Ibid., pp. 83-84.

27. Samuel Harry Popper, "Newark, N.J., 1870-1910: Chapters in the Evolution of an American Metropolis" (Unpublished Ph.D. diss., New York University, 1952), pp. 100-2, 120-1; Austin J. Tobin, "The Meadows as a Transportation Hub," *Newark Commerce: Newark Association of Commerce and Industry, Newark, N.J.*, Vol. VII, No. 5 (Nov. 1962), 25-26.

28. *Newark Evening News*, May 4, 1889.

29. Rankin, *Sketches of Early Newark*, p. 85.

30. Ibid., p. 84.

31. Popper, "Newark," pp. 100-2, 120-1; Rankin, *Sketches of Early Newark*, p. 85.

32. Headlee, *The Mosquitoes of New Jersey*, p. 3; Cowen, *Medicine and Health in New Jersey*, pp. 165-6.

33. Cowen, *Medicine and Health in New Jersey*, p. 165.

34. *Sunday Call*, Sept. 5, 1897.

35. Cowen, *Medicine and Health in New Jersey*, pp. 166-7; Headlee, *The Mosquitoes of New Jersey*, pp. 260-4; *Newark Evening News*, July 3,

1903; Smith, *Report of the New Jersey State Experimental Agricultural Station,* pp. 370-5.

36. Cowen, *Medicine and Health in New Jersey,* pp. 166-7; *NJMEA Proceedings, 1915,* p. 11.

37. *Newark Annual Reports, 1905, Board of Health,* p. 724, *1906,* p. 705, *1908,* p. 292, *1909,* p. 309, *1910,* pp. 450-5, *1911,* pp. 477-9; *Newark Evening News,* Aug. 26, 1908.

38. Headlee, *The Mosquitoes of New Jersey,* p. 266; *Newark Evening News,* July 18, 25, 1903; *NJMEA Proceedings, 1915,* pp. 11-12.

39. Cowen, *Medicine and Health in New Jersey,* p. 167.

40. Ibid., p. 168.

41. *Sunday Call,* July 16, 1911; *Newark Evening News,* August 26, 1908, June 28, Dec. 6, 1911; *NJMEA Proceedings, 1915,* p. 12.

42. Cowen, *Medicine and Health in New Jersey,* p. 168; *ARNJBH, 1912,* p. 28.

43. *NJMEA Proceedings, 1915,* pp. 13, 108-9; *ARNJBH, 1912,* p. 29.

44. *ARECMEC, 1912-1913,* pp. 7-12, 18; *ARNJBH, 1912,* p. 30.

45. *ARECMEC, 1914-1915,* pp. 11-12.

46. Ibid., *1912-1913,* pp. 13-15, 34-35.

47. Ibid., *1914-1915,* pp. 8, 19-21. A pumping station was built on the Newark meadows in 1887 to help rid the area of sewage.

48. Joseph Fulford Fulsom, *The Municipalities of Essex County, New Jersey: 1666-1924* (4 vols.; New York: The Lewis Historical Publishing Co., Inc., 1925), II, 457-8.

49. Cunningham, *Newark,* pp. 246-8, 255-6.

50. *ARECMEC, 1917-1918,* p. 1.

51. *NJMEA Proceedings, 1918,* p. 49.

52. Ibid., *1914,* pp. 10-12.

53. *ARECMEC, 1917-1918,* p. 3; *Newark Evening News,* Nov. 23, 1915.

54. *ARECMEC, 1923-1924.*

55. Ibid.

56. Below, Appendix.

57. *NJMEA Proceedings, 1914,* pp. 10-12.

58. Cowen, *Medicine and Health in New Jersey,* pp. 168-9: Ibrahim Elsammak, "Newark's 3,000 Meadow Acres," *Newark Commerce: Newark Association of Commerce and Industry,* Newark, N.J., VII, No. 5 (Nov. 1962), 12-13, 42.

7

Milk Reform

Dr. Coit was worried. The infant's intestinal ailment was getting worse and his mother, unable to breast feed, could not find a safe, wholesome milk. Coit's interest in the case was decidedly personal, for the patient was his firstborn infant son.[1]

As his son's life slipped away, Coit tried desperately to find a good quality milk. In the course of his search he observed the unsanitary conditions under which milk was produced in the late nineteenth century.

Cows were confined in poorly lighted, badly ventilated, unclean barns, or in muddy enclosures littered at times with knee-deep compost through which the animals were compelled to wade. Filth became encrusted on their flanks and udders which was not removed before milking. Farm workers with unclean hands and clothing milked the cows. No facilities were available for proper washing and sterilization of milk utensils, and frequently they were merely rinsed in some nearby stream or open body of stagnant water. Cooling of the milk was partially done, if at all, and the health condition of the cow or of the worker was given no consideration.[2]

The conditions uncovered by Coit spotlighted a nationwide crisis. Milk was a public health disaster area.[3] Shaken by his discoveries, Coit began a fight for clean milk, a crusade which at first he waged almost single-handed and which was to occupy him for the rest of his life.

Milk is man's most important food. It is the natural food of babies—rich in proteins and vitamins, high in calcium, easily digested, inexpensive, and capable of a great variety of modifications.[4]

While good milk has done more than any other single food to obtain and maintain health, bad milk was formerly responsible for more sickness and death than perhaps all other foods combined.[5]

Milk is dangerous because it spoils rapidly and is easily contaminated. Bacteria in unchilled milk will multiply a thousand- or a millionfold in a matter of hours. Compounding the danger, it is nearly impossible to keep milk sterile. Some bacteria are passed through the udder of the cow, and as soon as the milk leaves the teat it is subject to contamination by nearly every object it touches. Stable dust, filthy hands, dirty pails, and unwashed bottles are just a few of the vehicles by which milk may become tainted. Moreoever, unlike other foods, impurity in milk can not be detected by its appearance. A rich white-looking and sweet-tasting milk could nevertheless be dangerous.[6]

Milk-borne diseases include: tuberculosis, typhoid and paratyphoid fevers, diphtheria, gastroenteritis, scarlet fever, septic sore throat, and undulant fever. Though a few of these diseases (tuberculosis, septic sore throat, and undulant fever) may be transmitted through infection of the udders, milk usually becomes infected through exposure to a diseased person.[7] United States Public Health Bulletin No. 56, *Milk and its Relation to the Public Health,* listed some five hundred milk-borne epidemics between 1880 and 1907.[8]

Milk need not contain pathogenic microorganisms to be harmful. Consumption of milk high in bacteria or low in butter fat, milk solids, and other nutrients contributes to intestinal and constitutional ailments in children. Infants raised on impoverished milk suffer from diarrhea and poor bone development. Poor milk was thus an important factor in the high infant mortality rates of the late nineteenth and early twentieth centuries.[9]

The first groping steps toward a policy of government protection of the milk supply were taken in the 1870s in an attempt to prevent the sale of adulterated milk. Doctoring of milk was a common practice. Dairymen and retailers "skimmed" the cream from the milk and "watered" it. Through feats of alchemy involving the use of chemical preservatives such as sodium carbonate, potassium nitrate, tumeric, annatto, caramel, salt, and borax, milk that was thin, bluish, and watery became rich, white, and creamy. The preservatives also hid acid fermentation and delayed curdling.[10]

The agitation of public health officials, physicians, and the state board of agriculture led in 1875 to the enactment of New Jersey's first milk code The law prohibited the sale of "impure, adulterated or unwholesome milk" and milk from cows kept "in a crowded or unhealthy condition " or fed distillery wastes or decayed nutrients. As was typical of early regulatory milk legislation, the law was unenforceable. No standards of purity were specified and prosecution was dependent upon privately initiated legal action.[11]

In the next few years a number of trade measures were enacted on behalf of the milk industry to curb unfair competition among dealers. In 1878 a law providing for the labeling of skimmed milk was passed, and in 1880 a State Milk Inspector was appointed.[12] In 1881 the meaning of the term "adulterated milk" was broadened to include milk that had been tampered with in any way, and in 1882 the sale of milk containing less than 12 percent milk solids was forbidden.[13]

The sale of "watered" and "skimmed" milk cost Newark consumers about $60,000 annually.[14] To eliminate this fraud, the State Milk Inspector began to subject milk sold by retailers to a lactometer test.[15] The lactometer, however, only indicated the specific gravity of the fluid and not its composition. Hence by first removing the lighter cream from the milk and then adding the heavier water, vendors could adulterate milk without detection.[16] In 1889 the State Dairy Commissioner, who in 1885 had been assigned the duties of the State Milk Inspector, conceded he had been unsuccessful in preventing the sale of "skimmed" milk and the tests were discontinued. Subsequently the policing of municipal milk supplies was made a local responsibility.[17]

A state commission to investigate cases of bovine tuberculosis was established in 1894. The commission was authorized to examine sickly cows upon application of the cow's owner, the New Jersey Board of Health, or the State Dairy Commissioner, but could not act of its own volition. The commission members were appointed by the president of the state board of agriculture.

Both the commission and the state board of agriculture were dominated by spokesmen for the dairy industry, who adopted the "public be damned" attitude of late nineteenth-century plutocrats. In this spirit they opposed the compulsory tuberculin testing of cattle as a "radical" measure that would endanger the dairy industry. They further counseled against the imposition of "impossible" sanitary standards and stated that consumers were more at fault for poor milk than dairymen. High prices, they argued, and not coercive legislation, would guarantee pure, wholesome milk.[18]

Attempts at regulating the milk supply were initially more concerned with the consumer's pocketbook than his health. But as the distance between city and country grew, citizens became aware that the milk they consumed might be dangerous. The identification of pathogenic germs in the late nineteenth century focused attention on the fact that bacteria thrive in milk. As early as 1873, Abraham Jacobi, the father of American pediatrics, advised mothers to "boil the milk until you see the bubbles." A crusade for safe, wholesome milk developed in the first decade of the twentieth century. One of the first men to give voice to the need for an improved milk supply was a Newarker, Dr. Henry Leber Coit, "the Father of Clean Milk."

Coit, the son of a Methodist clergyman, was born March 16, 1854. After graduating with honors from the College of Pharmacy in New York, Coit worked briefly as a chemist for a commercial firm. With the money he saved he was able to attend Columbia's renowned College of Physicians and Surgeons. In 1884 he began practicing medicine as a general practitioner in Newark but soon limited his work to pediatrics. In the course of treating infants Coit became concerned about the quality of the commercial milk available to mothers who could not nurse their young. Following the death of his infant son in 1888, Coit set out on a path that would win him national and international acclaim as the originator of certified milk.[19]

The high toll of infant fatalities that resulted from unsanitary dairy conditions deeply troubled Coit.[20] Newark's infant mortality rate for 1889 was nearly 20 percent. Infant deaths constituted more than 25 percent of the city's entire mortality.[21] Four years later Coit was to write to his sister: "Five thousand little graves were dug last year in Philadelphia alone that were unnecessary and might have been avoided had the victims been provided with good milk."[22]

Deciding that something had to be done, during the years 1889-1893 Coit devoted whatever spare time he could find to visiting dairies and meeting with dairymen. In 1890 he asked the New Jersey State Medical Society to make an investigation into the relationship between the high infant mortality rates in urban communities and the milk supply, and was named chairman of a committee that reported on abuses in the production and sale of cow's milk. Coit now attempted to secure a better general milk supply through legislation but was thwarted by the opposition of "powerful commercial interests." Dairying was already a large industry in New Jersey and a force to be reckoned with in state politics.[24]

Failing to secure legislative relief, in January 1893, in a paper read before the Practitioner's Club of Newark, the city's leading medical fraternity, Coit proposed the formation of a medical milk commission. It would be composed of physicians serving without pay, who would supervise and certify the dairy production of a high-grade milk. A contract would give the commission control over the location and character of the land, the construction of buildings, the water supply, the health and breeding of the dairy stock, the housing and care of the cows, the collection, cooling, and preparation for shipment of the milk, and its bottling and transportation. Bacteriologists and chemists engaged to inspect the dairies would have their fees paid by the dairy owner. In return, the dairy owner would be allowed to affix the label "certified" to his product and thus could hope to command a higher price. Not intended for mass market consumption, the milk would be used primarily by infants and the sick, whom the contract would specify as "preferred purchasers."[25]

As the plan entailed a large capital outlay, Coit was lucky to find an idealistic dairyman, Stephen Francisco, the proprietor of Fairfield Dairy in Caldwell, New Jersey, who was willing to take the risks involved. Legislative consent was given to the creation of the Essex County Medical Milk Commission, and on May 19, 1893, a contract was signed with the Fairfield Dairy. On June 14, 1893, the first instrument of certification was issued.[26] Coit wrote at this time: "I expect within five years to reduce the death rate in Newark 40 or 50 per cent." ". . . what is best of all," added Coit, prophetically, "the scheme is likely . . . to revolutionize the entire milk business."[27]

The duties of the Medical Milk Commission were twofold: 1) to establish clinical standards of purity for cow's milk—physical, chemical, and bacteriological yardsticks for measuring milk's cleanliness, nutritive value, and freedom from contamination; and 2) to insure compliance with these standards and with the other requirements and regulations of the commission through periodic investigations. During these inspections sanitary conditions were evaluated, herds were tested for tuberculosis, employees were examined for communicable diseases, and chemical and bacteriological examinations of the milk were made.[28]

The commission met regularly to discuss new dairy methods. Very little escaped the commission's attention; not even something so minor as what to do with the cow's tail during milking was overlooked. Out of these discussions came many innovations in dairying, including grooming of cows, screening, immediate cooling and early bottling of the milk, and medical supervision of herds and employees.[29]

Within a few years the work of the Essex County Medical Milk Commission was known nationally. Articles on Coit's work appeared in medical journals and the press. Coit himself was the author of some forty-odd treatises on milk, infant feeding, pediatrics, and related subjects, and was in constant demand as a lecturer. By 1906 there were twenty-seven medical milk commissions in the United States, and in 1907 a national organization, The American Association of Medical Milk Commissions, was formed. From America the idea spread to Europe. In 1911 a committee composed of the Assistant Surgeon General, Coit, and another physician was appointed to prepare a code of working methods and regulations to serve as a guide for the commissions.[30]

At the instigation of Coit, in 1909 a bill was passed providing for the incorporation of medical milk commissions in New Jersey. Medical milk commissions were empowered to enter into agreements with dairymen for production of certified milk, provided their requirements met the standards set by the American Association of Medical Milk Commissions. The New Jersey Board of Health was made responsible for enforcing the act. Similar laws passed in other states helped to insure the character and good name of certified milk.[31]

In Essex County, the home of the movement, the market for certified milk expanded from one delivery in one city in 1893 to twenty-two deliveries in twenty-seven cities and townships in 1915. About 3 percent of the milk sold in Newark in 1907 was certified. When local milk dealers surreptitiously began placing the words "certified milk" on their wagons and milk, Coit and Francisco were forced to apply for a copyright. The Fairfield Dairy shared in the success of the Essex County Medical Milk Commission. In 1893 the dairy owned 100 acres of land and 9 cows, and had a daily productive capacity of 100 quarts of milk. By 1923 it possessed 1000 acres and 654 cows, and had a daily productive capacity of 6,500 quarts, of which 2,990 were certified.[32]

Certified milk had two serious drawbacks: 1) it was expensive—12 to 20¢ per quart—nearly double the price of commercial grades; and 2) it was raw milk and hence potentially dangerous. In time certified milk was replaced by pasteurized milk, and the regulatory and supervisory work of the medical milk commission was assumed by the state.[33]

Nevertheless, Coit's contribution was a lasting one. Medical milk commissions were responsible for the introduction of the covered milk pail, the milk utensil sterilizer, and the application of bacteriology to the safeguarding of milk. It was a medical milk commission that first required the tuberculin testing of herds, and it was agitation on the part of the commissions that led the United States Government to assume responsibility for the implementation of this reform.[34] Of greater consequence than any new techniques developed, the publicity attending the certified milk movement awakened interest in the whole subject of milk reform and infant and child welfare. "Every community possessing a Milk Commission," wrote Dr. Otto P. Grier, the secretary and a later president of the American Association of Medical Milk Commissions,

> has been benefited by a better understanding of and a deeper interest in the clean milk movement and child welfare work. In most instances the Commission has borne not only the burden of pure milk propaganda, but has definitely effected an improvement in the administration of public health matters.[35]

Though certified milk never constituted a very large percentage of the total milk supply, the high standards advanced by the commissions provided a goal for reformers and led to a general improvement in dairy inspection and milk sanitation. Moreover, certified milk afforded safe raw milk at a time when raw milk and mother's milk were considered the only suitable foods for infants, and much of the commercial milk supply, both raw and pasteurized, was suspect. Finally, the death rate among infants raised on certified milk was markedly lower than for those weaned on milk sold to the general public.[36]

Pasteurization is a process whereby milk is made safe and fermentation retarded through heating. The milk is heated to a temperature below the boiling point for a specified period of time, and then rapidly cooled. Pasteurization destroys the harmful bacteria in milk without impairing its taste and nutritional value. "Next to water purification, pasteurization is the most important single preventive measure in the field of sanitation."[37] The idea of pasteurizing milk was suggested by the low temperatures used by Pasteur in heating wine and beer. In 1892 Nathan Straus, a department store owner and philanthropist, established milk stations in the tenement districts of New York City, where pasteurized milk was sold for cost or given away free to indigent children. A pasteurizing plant installed by Straus in a foundling hospital on Randalls Island in New York helped bring about an amazing 65 percent decline in the institution's infant mortality rate.

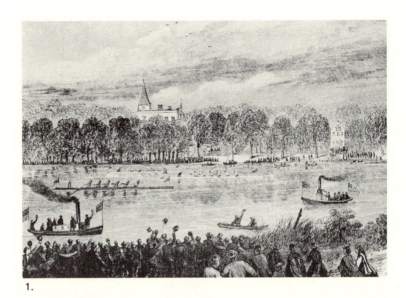

1.

"The First New Jersey State Rowing Regatta, on the Passaic River, at Newark, N.J., Saturday, Oct. 10th—From Sketch by Jas. E. Taylor." Harper's Weekly, 1868. Collections of the New Jersey Historical Society.

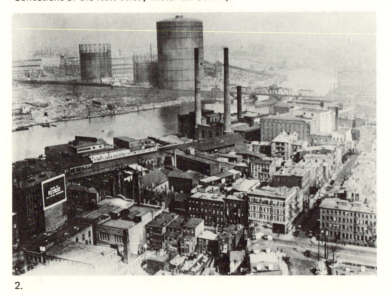

2.

The Passaic River despoiled, a victim of industrialization. 1926. Courtesy of the Newark Public Library.

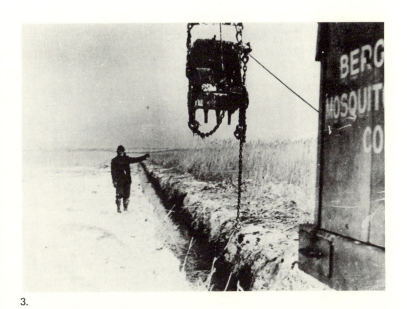

3.

Winter construction of a drainage ditch in the Newark salt meadows. Date unknown.
Courtesy of the Newark Public Library.

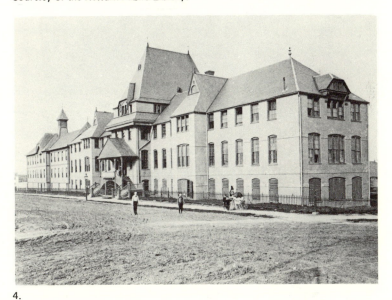

4.

Newark City Hospital. 1892. Courtesy of the Newark Public Library.

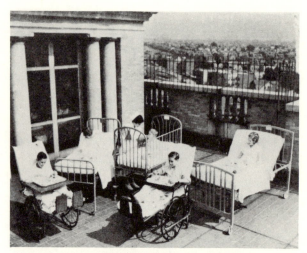

MEAL TIME on children's sun deck at Beth Israel Hospital.

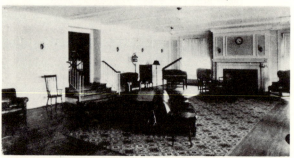

RECEPTION ROOM of nurses' home at Beth Israel Hospital.

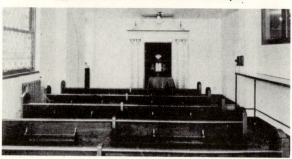

5.

Scenes at Beth Israel Hospital. Date unknown. Courtesy of the Newark Public Library.

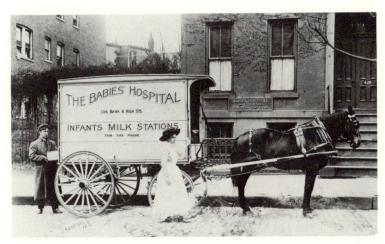

6.

Safe, wholesome milk was made available to the infants of indigent parents through milk stations established by private philanthropy and by the government. Date unknown. Courtesy of the Newark Public Library.

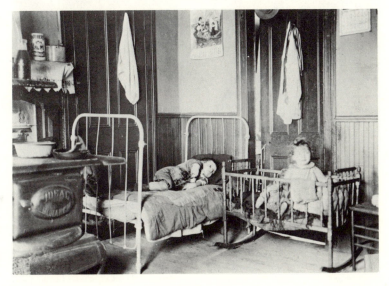

7.

Tenement living conditions were detrimental to their inhabitants' health and morals. Date unknown. Courtesy of the Newark Public Library.

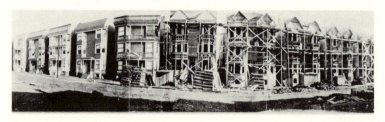

8.

Housing constructed under the provisions of the New Jersey Tenement House Law of 1904 afforded a few Newarkers their first decent housing, N.J., *Report of the Board of Tenement House Supervision, 1905.*

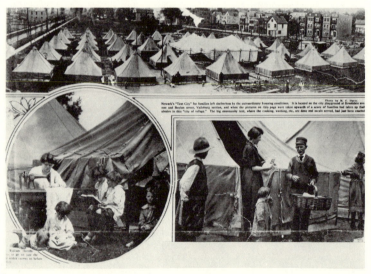

9.

Homeless victims of the October 5, 1918 munitions plant explosion in Morgan, New Jersey, were provided a temporary shelter in Newark, where housing was already in short supply as a result of World War I. The makeshift housing afforded the Morgan refugees and the ramshackle accommodation provided Southern Negro migrants, who came to Newark seeking war work, left these groups defenseless before the fury of the 1918 influenza epidemic.

Nevertheless, pasteurization did not win immediate approbation. Pediatricians objected to it on the grounds that it impaired digestability and destroyed necessary proteins and enzymes; some feared it would lead to scurvy. Advocates of certified milk were concerned that pasteurization would be used to redeem dirty, impoverished milk. Adoption of pasteurization was also delayed by the backward state of pasteurization technology. There was no agreed-upon method of pasteurizing milk, and commercial pasteurization machinery was unreliable. By 1900 a number of milk dealers in large metropolitan areas were using pasteurization to prevent souring, but it was done surreptitiously, since pasteurization did not have the approval of the majority of public health authorities.[38]

At first Coit endorsed pasteurization, calling it "one of the most important steps taken by preventive medical science in recent years."[39] Before establishing his milk stations, Straus had corresponded with Coit and had asked his help in establishing the depots. Coit, who at the time was busy formulating his own solution to the milk problem, provided Straus with a letter of introduction to Dr. R. G. Freeman, the leading American advocate of pasteurization.[40]

Later Coit reversed himself and raised the objection that the marketing of inferior milk redeemed by pasteurization would undermine the dairy methods and standards so painstakingly arrived at by the medical milk commissions. Coit further believed commercial pasteurization was intrinsically unsafe. Coit did not oppose pasteurization when performed at home or in milk depots at the behest of a physician and under medical supervision.[41] When a movement developed around 1910 for the compulsory pasteurization of municipal milk supplies, the medical milk commissions formed the vanguard of the opposition.[42] Still later Coit came to believe that pasteurization destroyed the vitamins in milk and that pasteurized milk was therefore unsuited for infant use.[43]

In the meantime, the milk reform movement had progressed along a broad front as a result of technical, scientific, and medical advances. In 1908 Milton J. Rosenau, Professor of Preventive Medicine at Harvard University, showed that pasteurization could be performed without causing deleterious chemical changes by heating milk to a temperature of 60°C. for twenty minutes. In 1910 the American Public Health Association devised standard methods for the bacteriological testing of milk. About the same time, the dairy scorecard was widely adopted as the best means of grading the sanitary condition of dairies. In addition, the dairy scorecard showed dairymen that the production of safe, wholesome milk need not be expensive. Thus in 1910 Dr. Charles E. North of New York City demonstrated that by strictly adhering to recognized sanitary procedures dairymen who could not afford the expensive machinery used by certified dealers could produce a high quality milk at a cost of only one cent above the market price of most commercial grades.[44] From this point on reasonably clean milk made safe by pasteurization began to gain at the expense of certified milk. This was especially the case after a serious epidemic of septic sore throat in Boston in 1910 was traced to use of raw milk from a "model" dairy.[45] in 1911 a national commission on milk standards proposed a system of milk grading based on the sanitary care attending milk's production and its bacterial count. The plan was endorsed by the American Public Health Association and the United States Public Health Service.[46] In 1912 New York City took the initiative in implementing the commission's recommendations by requiring the pasteurization of all milk used for drinking purposes, except for raw milk of the highest quality, and by adopting a grading system.[47]

Coit's prominence in the movement notwithstanding, milk reform received little attention in Newark prior to 1911. In 1882 the board of health detailed an inspector to assist in enforcing the state milk code. As of 1894 the board still employed only one milk inspector—and his work was singularly unsuccessful.[48]

In 1902 a municipal milk ordinance was passed authorizing the board of health to license vendors. Milk dealers were required to submit the names of their suppliers and customers and were prohibited from selling adulterated milk and milk from diseased cows or from dairies where unsanitary conditions prevailed or communicable diseases were present. Unfortunately, nearly all of the milk consumed in Newark was produced outside the city. Lacking the authority and the money to inspect out-of-city dairies, the board of health was powerless to enforce the code. The licensing provisions of the statute soon became little more than a means of raising revenue.[49]

In 1906 the board of health, which had begun the bacteriological examination of the milk supply, reported the existence of high bacteria counts, the result of years of unconscionable neglect on the part of the board and the city.[50] Even low bacterial counts, however, fail to provide foolproof protection if other control measures are not in effect. In 1906 a milk-borne epidemic of typhoid fever occurred. When it was discovered that over 85 percent of the victims received their milk from one source, the indicated milk was tested repeatedly, but was "found to be as good, if not a little better than the average." Inspectors were sent to investigate the company's milkshed and

> several cases of typhoid fever were discovered, some even in the household of farmers who were delivering milk to the collection depot of the milk company, where it was mixed with a larger quantity of milk from other sources, the resulting mixture being of passable quality.[51]

As a result of this incident the bacteriologist of the board of health proposed the pasteurization of all milk not "clearly above suspicion."[52] His suggestion fell on deaf ears. The board of health was lethargic and would not act unless goaded.

A newspaper campaign for milk reform finally shook the board of health from its apathy. Throughout most of 1911 and 1912 a series of articles appeared in the *Newark Evening News* showing that the city's health was being imperiled by the board's failure to protect the milk supply. The lead article had as its starting point the city's excessive infant mortality. A farmer who lost as large a percentage of his livestock, commented Coit, would be bankrupt. The *News* announced that, as the chances of survival of most infants were directly dependent upon the purity of store-bought milk, it had: 1) purchased milk from the city's retail outlets; 2) observed the conditions under which it was dispensed; and 3) submitted the milk to laboratory analysis.[53]

In one store visited by the *Newark Evening News* the milk was obtained from cows housed in adjoining sheds. The sheds had no ventilation and were in semidarkness. The bodies of the cows were smeared with manure and the floors were covered with dirt. During the winter, the cows were fed household slops and brewery grains. When the weather turned warm, the cows were turned loose on vacant lots to feed on garbage. The bacterial count of the milk was over 7 million bacteria per cubic centimeter—nor was this atypical. Milk with a bacterial count of more than 6.5 million bacteria per cubic centimeter was being sold in large sections of Newark and few samples taken anywhere in the city fell below 1 million bacteria per cubic centimeter, the "very greatest number permitted by any bacterial standard anywhere suggested."[54]

Other revelations followed. As many customers could not afford to pay the extra two cents, only about half of the milk sold in Newark was bottled. The remainder was dipped from cans and poured into containers. Frequent opening of the cans exposed the milk to dirt and dust. The hands of the man doing the ladling went unwashed and the dipping utensils were not sterilized. No effort was made to chill the milk, and in one instance the milk can was situated near a stove. In about one-third of the stores the proprietor and his family lived on the premises.[55]

On February 28 the health officer promised to institute reforms. At the time the board of health employed two milk inspectors to look after 875 stores and 325 wagons. On March 14, the *News* commented editorially. Calling the conditions it had found "intolerable in an enlightened city," the *News* asked for closer supervision of the retail milk trade, new laws, more vigorous enforcement of existing statutes, an increase in the number of milk inspectors, and establishment of bacterial standards for milk.[56]

A few weeks later by resolution of the board of health the standard of milk cleanliness was fixed at 500,000 bacteria per cubic centimeter. The board also stated that it would publicly record the names of milk dealers regularly selling milk with less than 100,000 bacteria per cubic centimeter in a "Roll of Honor." Furthermore, it had revoked the licenses of nearly a dozen dealers.[57]

Stopgap measures proved ineffectual, and on June 15 the *News* reported there was little improvement in the milk situation. "The plain fact is," wrote the editor, "that Newark is almost without equipment for handling the milk problem." Not satisfied with the progress made during the summer months in September the *News* endorsed a plea made by the subcommittee on health of the Essex County Public Welfare Committee for establishing an independent milk division within the health department.[58]

In December 1911 the *News* shifted its attention to the dairies supplying Newark with milk. The first story was headlined: "Revolting Conditions in Dairies Discovered at Twenty Places Almost Beyond Belief." Among the most appalling conditions uncovered at the dairies, which were located just outside the city, were the practice of milking sick cows, the use of filthy rags to strain the milk, and the presence of manure, garbage, and dead animals heaped against the sheds. Not a single dairy met the minimum standards established by the United States Government Dairy Scorecard. Few dairies were regularly inspected by either the city or the state; one dairy had not been investigated in six years. Dairy inspection, the *News* concluded, was a farce.[59]

Efforts to reform the conditions under which milk was produced were resisted by the dairy industry. Use of the tuberculin test was opposed because little or no state compensation was given farmers for the loss of diseased cows.[60] Farm groups protested that the expense of complying with tough dairy laws would drive the small dairyman out of business, force prices up, and result in a milk shortage. In a series of editorials the *News* endeavored to assuage the fears of the dairy farmer.[61] Dirt, dust, and heat, it was argued, were the most important factors in producing high bacterial counts. Since the United States Government Dairy Score-card allotted sixty points for cleanliness and only forty points for equipment, and because there was little expense involved in using hot water, soap, whitewash, and ice, the small farmer need not fear stringent government regulations. Indeed, better dairy sanitation would result in healthier cows, a higher grade of milk, and larger milk output. Even if the objections of dairy farmers had substance, they would be of no consequence, for

> one baby poisoned by dirty milk represents a loss to society besides which the fancied savings effected by filthy methods in all the dirty dairies of the country are trivial in comparison.[62]

Throughout the remainder of 1911 and most of 1912 the *News* continued its campaign for milk reform. In addition to reporting the findings of its investigations, the presses of the *News* poured forth a stream of articles on virtually every aspect of the milk question, including bovine tuberculosis and the tuberculin testing of cows, pasteurization, the care of milk in the home, and milk bottling.[63]

The seeds planted by the *News* bore their first fruits in 1912. In January 1912 the board of health announced it would investigate all dairies supplying Newark with milk. Dairies which failed in two successive tests to attain a mark of 60 percent on the United States Government Dairy Scorecard would be prohibited from marketing milk in Newark. The number of milk inspectors was doubled, and a food and drug committee was established within the department.[64] Thus the inspection and scoring of dairies was begun. In the first year 1,115 dairies, 18 creameries, and 80 bottling plants were visited.[65] The *News* reported an almost 100 percent improvement in the sanitary state of shops and cowbarns within the city.[66] Rural dairies, however, failed to show any improvement.[67]

On April 29, 1913, a special meeting of the Essex County Medical Society was convened in response to warnings of the United States Public

Health Service that communicable diseases were being spread by dairy products other than milk. Consumers could shield themselves against the worst consequences of tainted milk by using home pasteurizers or by boiling the milk, but obviously could not afford themselves the same protection when consuming ice cream, butter, or cheese.[68] The society was alarmed because most of Essex County's milk products were not

TABLE 3

Daily Milk Consumption in Newark, 1913

Total consumption	118,000	quarts
Amount sold raw	54,000	"
Amount sold pasteurized	64,000	"
Amount brought in by railroads	91,750	"
Amount brought in from suburbs	22,000	"
Amount produced in city	4,250	"
Number of wagons selling milk	400	"
Number of stores selling milk	925	"

SOURCE: Newark Annual Reports,
1913, Board of Health, pp.969-70

pasteurized and only 2 percent of its milk was obtained from tuberculin-tested cows.[69] Recognizing that inspection alone had not provided adequate protection and probably never would, the society recommended that "outside of a very limited amount of inspected and certified milk," all market milk be pasteurized. At this time, of course, many prominent Newark physicians were opposed to compulsory pasteurization.[70] The society also created a permanent committee to lobby for changes in the state's milk laws.[71]

A little over a month later the Russell Sage Foundation's report on the department of health was released. The report lambasted the board of health for its belated and feeble attempts to regulate the milk supply. Analysis of the milk samples taken in 1912, the report stated, presented incontrovertible evidence that Newark was confronted with a milk crisis.[72]

As a result of the Russell Sage Foundation report, a comprehensive milk ordinance embracing most of the provisions of the New York City code of 1912 was adopted by Newark in December 1913. One provision required all milk marketed in Newark to be classified according to sanitary conditions of production and bacterial count into one of five grades:

1. Certified   Milk produced under the supervision of the Essex County Medical Milk Commission and containing less than 10,000 bacteria per cubic centimeter.

2. Grade A, Raw   Milk produced from tuberculin-tested cows on dairies scoring at least 65 percent on the United States Government Dairy Scorecard and containing not more than 100,000 bacteria per cubic centimeter.

3. Grade A, Pasteurized   Milk produced on dairies scoring at least 40 percent on the United States Government Dairy Scorecard and containing not more than 200,000 bacteria per cubic centimeter before pasteurization, and 30,000 bacteria per cubic centimeter after pasteurization.

4. Grade B, Pasteurized   Milk produced on dairies scoring at least 40 percent on the United States Government Dairy Scorecard, and containing not more than 1 million bacteria per cubic centimeter before pasteurization, and 50,000 bacteria per cubic centimeter after pasteurization.

5. Grade C Milk used for cooking or industrial purposes; to be sold only in bulk, and to be heated prior to sale to a temperature of 200°F. for a period of two minutes.

Another section forbade the sale of milk stored at a temperature of more than 50°F. or that failed a sediment test (a test to determine the presence of visible dirt by filtering a pint of milk through a disc of absorbent cotton one inch in diameter).[73] Adulterated milk was defined as milk to which anything had been either added or removed. The sale of milk containing less than 11½ percent milk solids or 3 percent fat was prohibited.

Still other articles of the law dealt with bottling and the medical supervision of dairy herds. The sale of loose milk, except upon permit of the board of health, was prohibited in stores after September 1, 1915. Dairymen were compelled to remove diseased cows and to submit their herds to yearly physical examinations by a veterinarian approved by the board of health. In addition, they were forbidden to add unexamined cows to tuberculin-tested herds. Finally, the board of health was given the power to regulate the sale of cream, condensed milk, buttermilk, and skim milk.[74]

The law was not popular with dairymen and would require strict enforcement to be effective. In 1914 a shortage of money prevented the board of health from inspecting outlying creameries and dairies.[75] In contrast to the board of health, which claimed a significant improvement,[76] the *Newark Evening News* reported that Newark was still behind other municipalities in milk inspection.[77]

Milk inspection proceeded at a snail's pace until the reorganization of the board of health in 1915. Under new leadership, the board began a vigorous campaign to improve the milk supply. Over five times as many dairies were inspected in 1915 as in 1913, and over twice as many samples were taken as in the previous year. New laboratory equipment was ordered and testing was begun to determine the presence of pus and streptococci.[78] As a rejoinder to criticism made of its techniques of milk analysis,[79] the board announced that all bacteriological testing was being done in accordance with the methods established by the American Public Health Association.[80]

The New Jersey Bovine Tuberculosis Commission endeavored to redress the grievances of the dairy industry by securing partial state indemnity for destroyed cows and by requiring the tuberculin examination of imported dairy cows and breeding cattle. When diseased cattle continued to be dumped in New Jersey, the responsibility for the inspection of imported cattle was shifted from the veterinarians and officials of the exporting states to the New Jersey Department of Agriculture. In 1918

New Jersey adopted the accredited herd plan of the United States Government for the control and eradication of bovine tuberculosis. The plan
requires the tuberculin testing of all milch cows and the slaughtering of
positive reactors. Under this plan only milk produced by tuberculin-tested
herds can be sold to the public. In line with the recommendations of the
United States Bureau of Animal Husbandry, animals slaughtered because
of a positive tuberculin reaction, but not judged unfit for human consumption, were permitted to be sold for beef.[81]

Other improvements in milk inspection were also realized. The board
of health gained the right to supervise the operation of pasteurizing plants,
and the sale of unbottled milk was prohibited. Stringent regulations made
it difficult for producers of raw milk to avoid compulsory pasteurization
so that by 1920, 80 percent of the milk consumed in Newark was
pasteurized.[82]

Dairy inspection was a more difficult task. The milk supply was drawn
from over 3,000 dairies at distances from Newark of up to 400 miles. Lack
of funds prevented the board of health from inspecting dairies beyond a
fifty-mile radius. Consequently, many of the dairies supplying Newark
with milk, nearly all of it pasteurized milk shipped in by railroad, escaped
inspection.[83]

By the end of 1918 the board of health had achieved most of the goals
sought by milk reformers: dairy inspection, pasteurization, bottling, grading,
and the tuberculin testing of cows. Newark at long last had moved alongside
other progressive cities in the regulation of its municipal milk supply.

NOTES

1. *Clean Milk: A Bi-Monthly Publication Issued by the Medical Milk
Commission of Essex County, N.J.*, IV, No. 2 (March 1923), National
Library of Medicine, Henry Leber Coit MSS.

2. *Certified Milk: Official Publication of American Association of
Medical Milk Commissions, Inc., and Certified Milk Producers of America,
Inc.*, XXIV, No. 8 (Aug. 1949), 2.

3. *Trans. MSNJ, 1892,* p. 77; New Jersey, State Board of Agriculture,
Annual Report, 1892-1893, pp. 150-1, *1897* pp. 153-4 (hereinafter
referred to as *ARNJBA*).

4. Milton J. Rosenau, *Preventive Medicine and Hygiene* (6th ed.; New
York: D. Appleton and Co., 1913), p. 752.

5. Ibid., p. 753.

6. Ibid., pp. 373-4.

7. Fred B. Rogers, *Help Bringers: Versatile Physicians of New Jersey* (New York: Vantage Press, Inc., 1961), p. 119; Charles Wilcocks, *Medical Advance, Public Health, and Social Evolution* (Oxford: Pergamon Press, 1965), p. 143.

8. Manfred J. Wasserman, "Henry L. Coit and the Certified Milk Movement in the Development of Modern Pediatrics," *Bulletin of the History of Medicine,* XLV, No. 4 (July-Aug. 1972), 360.

9. Henry Leber Coit, "The Causation of Disease by Milk and the Means of Prevention," *ARNJBH, 1894,* p. 370.

10. Blake McKelvey, *The Urbanization of America: 1860-1915* (New Brunswick, N.J.: Rutgers University Press, 1963), pp. 191-2; Rosenau, *Preventive Medicine,* 6th ed., p. 772.

11. Fred B. Rogers and A. Reasoner Sayre, *The Healing Art: A History of the Medical Society of New Jersey* (Trenton, N.J.: The Medical Society of New Jersey, 1966), p. 168; N.J., *Legislative Acts* (1875), pp. 58-59; *ARNJBH, 1880,* p. 230.

12. *ARNJBH, 1880,* p. 231; *ARNJBA, 1882-1883,* p. 143.

13. N.J., *Legislative Acts* (1881), pp. 283-5.

14. *Newark Annual Reports, 1882, Board of Health,* pp. 459-62.

15. Ibid., pp. 458-62, *1885,* p. 619.

16. *Trans. MSNJ, 1892,* pp. 79-80.

17. *Annual Report of the Board of Health, 1889,* p. 15; N.J., *Legislative Acts* (1901), pp. 186-99; *ARNJBH, 1897,* pp. 315-7; Henry L. Coit, *A Plan to Procure Cow's Milk Designed for Chemical Purposes: Paper Read before the Practitioner's Club, Newark, N.J., January, 1893;* N.J., *Report of the Dairy Commissioner for the Year 1893,* p. 11; *ARNJBA, 1893-1894,* pp. 236-7.

18. *ARNJBA, 1894-1895,* pp. 255-68, *1896-1897,* pp. 137-43, *1897,* p. 145, *1907,* p. 105, *1909,* pp. 73-74.

19. The American Association of Medical Milk Commissioners, *Proceedings of the Annual Conference, 1917,* 4th Sess., *Memorial Service to Doctor Henry L. Coit,* "The Father of Certified Milk," Coit MSS, Box 11 (hereinafter referred to as *AAMMC Proceedings*); *Clean Milk,* IV, No. 2 (March 1923), VII, No. 2 (March 1926). Other honors accrued to Coit. In 1896 he opened the second hospital in the United States devoted exclusively to infants, and in 1910 he founded and was the first president of the New Jersey Pediatrics Society. Rogers, *Versatile Physicians of New Jersey,* p. 122.

20. *Clean Milk,* IV, No. 2 (March 1923).

21. [Henry Leber] Coit, *The Feeding of Infants:* [Paper] *Read at a Meeting of the Practitioners Club, Newark, N.J.,* p. 1 (reprinted from *The Medical and Surgical Reporter,* June 7, 1890).

22. Letter, H. L. Coit to Carrie and Clarence, May 22, 1893, Coit MSS, Box 1.

23. Mildred V. Naylor, "Henry Leber Coit: A Biographical Sketch," *Bulletin of the History of Medicine,* XII, No. 2 (1942), 369; *Clean Milk,* II, No. 5 (September 1922); *Trans. MSNJ, 1892,* pp. 74-81; Wilson G. Smillie, *Public Health, Its Promise for the Future: A Chronicle of the Development of Public Health in the United States, 1607-1914* (New York: The Macmillan Co., 1955), pp. 353-4, 361. Coit, "A Plan to Procure Cow's Milk," pp. 10-11.

24. Rogers and Sayre, *The Healing Art,* p. 156.

25. Coit, "A Plan to Procure Cow's Milk," *passim.*

26. *AAMMC Proceedings, 1906;* [Henry Leber] Coit, *The Origin, Purpose and Working Methods of the Medical Milk Commission: Paper Read at a Meeting Held by the Pediatric Club of Baltimore, Maryland, May 31, 1903,* p. 1 (reprinted, from the *Maryland Medical Journal,* Aug. 1903).

27. Letter, H. L. Coit to Carrie and Clarence, May 22, 1893, Coit MSS, Box 1.

28. [Henry Leber] Coit, *Aperçu Historique du Développement pris aux États Unis par le Mouvement pour la Consommation du Lait Pur: . . . Discours Prononcé au Congrès International des Gouttes de Lait Bruxelles, 12 Septembre, 1907.*

29. T. W. Harvey, *Early Days of the Essex County Milk Commission* (n.p., 1925).

30. *Certified Milk,* XXIV, No. 8 (Aug. 1949), 3; Smillie, *Public Health, Its Promise for the Future,* p. 361; Harvey, *Early Days of the Essex County Milk Commission; Clean Milk,* V, No. 3 (May 1924).

31. *AAMMC Proceedings, 1911,* pp. 13-17; *1913,* pp. 11-12.

32. Ibid., *1907,* p. 36, *1911,* p. 13, *1915,* p. 12; *Clean Milk,* IV, No. 3 (May 1923).

33. "From Certification to Pasteurization," *American Journal of Public Health,* XLIV (1954), 929-30; Smillie, *Public Health, Its Promise for the Future,* p. 361.

34. *Certified Milk,* XXIV, No. 8 (August 1949), 3; *Clean Milk,* I, No. 1 (March 1916); Letter, H. L. Coit to Dr. T. N. Gray, April 2, 1913, Coit MSS, Box 4.

35. *AAMMC Proceedings, 1917,* "Memorial Service to Doctor Henry L. Coit," Coit MSS, Box 11.

36. Smillie, *Public Health, Its Promise for the Future*, p. 361; Rogers, *Versatile Physicians of New Jersey*, p. 122; *AAMMC Proceedings, 1907*, p. 36.

37. Rosenau, *Preventive Medicine*, 6th ed., p. 759.

38. Charles E. North, "Milk and its Relation to Public Health," *A Half Century of Public Health: Jubilee Historical Volume of the American Public Health Association*, ed. Mazÿck Porcher Ravenel (New York: American Public Health Association, 1921), pp. 238-42, 274-5; Smillie, *Public Health, Its Promise for the Future*, pp. 361-3; McKelvey, *Urbanization of America*, p. 152; Newark, Department of Public Health, *Monthly Bulletin*, N.S., Vol. III, No. 2 (Feb. 1920); *ARNJBH, 1908*, p. 85.

39. Coit, "The Causation of Disease by Milk," p. 373.

40. *Trans. MSNJ, 1902*, p. 93; *Clean Milk*, VII, No. 2 (March 1926).

41. Coit, *Aperçu Historique*, pp. 4-6, 9; letter, H. L. Coit to Dr. Furrer, Jan. 15, 1916, Coit MSS, Box 4.

42. Smillie, *Public Health, Its Promise for the Future*, pp. 362-3; letters, H. L. Coit to Dr. G. L. Lloyd Magruder, Jan. 4, 8, 1911; letter, Charles C. Carlin to H. L. Coit, Jan. 23, 1911; letter, H. L. Coit to R. C. Caskey, n.d., Coit MSS, Box 4.

43. *Minutes of the District Medical Society, County of Essex, State of New Jersey, 1816-1920*, "Report of the Standing Committee on Milk," VI (1916), 9-14 (hereinafter referred to as *Minutes, ECMS*).

44. North, "Milk," pp. 241, 251, 260, 265, 274, 283; Smillie, *Public Health, Its Promise for the Future*, pp. 361-3.

45. "From Certification to Pasteurization," p. 929; Smillie, *Public Health, Its Promise for the Future*, pp. 262-3.

46. North, "Milk," p. 287.

47. Ibid., p. 241.

48. *Newark Annual Reports, 1882, Board of Health*, pp. 458-60; *Annual Report of the Board of Health, 1894*, pp. 45-47.

49. Newark, *Revised Ordinances* (1902), "Relating to Milk," pp. 575-7; *Annual Report of the Board of Health, 1902*, p. 58.

50. *Newark Annual Reports, 1905, Board of Health*, pp. 729-30; 1906, p. 728.

51. Ibid., *1906*, pp. 729-30.

52. Ibid., p. 730.

53. *Newark Evening News*, Feb. 21, 1911.

54. Ibid., Feb. 22, 1911.

55. Ibid., Feb. 21, 23, June 15, 1911.

56. Ibid., Feb. 28, March 14, 1911.

57. Ibid., April 8, 1911.

58. Ibid., June 15, Sept. 18, 1911.

59. Ibid., Dec. 19, 21, 1911.

60. Rogers and Sayre, *The Healing Art,* pp. 159-60; *Newark Evening News,* April 19, 1913.

61. *Newark Evening News,* Jan. 6, 10, 12, 1912.

62. Ibid., Jan. 17, 1912.

63. Ibid., June 9, July 3, 19, 29, Aug. 11, 1911; Jan. 22, Feb. 15, March 15, 21, April 6, June 18, 28, July 6, Aug. 2, 3, 12, 14, Sept. 18, Oct. 9, 17, 21, 1912.

64. Ibid., Jan. 16, 1912.

65. *Newark Annual Reports, 1912, Board of Health,* pp. 351-2.

66. *Newark Evening News,* May 1, 1912. In 1913 the food and drug committee was given division status within the department.

67. Ibid., June 15, 1912.

68. [Henry Leber] Coit, *A Method of Gathering Statistics of Milk Borne Morbidity and Mortality: Presidential Address before the Second Annual Meeting of the American Association of Medical Milk Commissions* (Chicago, June 1908), p. 5; *Sunday Call,* Aug. 8, 1912.

69. *Newark Evening News,* July 19, 1911.

70. Ibid., March 10, 1911.

71. *Minutes, ECMS,* "Special Meeting of the Essex County Medical Society, April 29, 1913," p.v.

72. *Newark Evening News,* June 5, 1913.

73. The dirt consists mainly of cow feces. As the dirt left on the cotton constitutes "visible evidence," the sediment test is a highly effective educational device for alerting farmers to the need for sanitary care. *Newark Annual Reports, 1918, Board of Health,* pp. 247-9. See also Rosenau, *Preventive Medicine,* 6th ed., pp. 757, 782-3.

74. Newark, *Revised Ordinances* (1913), *Addenda,* pp. 21-41; *Newark Annual Reports, 1915, Board of Health,* pp. 1007-9.

75. *Newark Annual Reports, 1914, Board of Health,* pp. 552-3.

76. Ibid.

77. *Newark Evening News,* August 6, 1914; see also April 9, 1914.

78. The existence of pus and streptococci in milk indicates an inflammation of the udder and is a danger sign of an impending outbreak of septic sore throat.

79. *Newark Evening News,* June 5, 1913, Dec. 12, 1914.

80. *Newark Annual Reports, 1915, Board of Health,* pp. 1012, 1018, 1025-31; North, "Milk," pp. 244-5.

81. *ARNJBA, 1894-1895,* pp. 255-68, *1897,* p. 152, *1900-1901,* p. 211, *1904,* p. 202, *1908,* pp. 56-57, 60, *1909,* p. 74, *1911,* pp. 69-71,

108-9, 139, 164-6; N.J., Department of Agriculture, *Annual Report, 1916-1917*, p. 311, *1918-1919*, p. 55.

82. *Newark Annual Reports, 1915, Board of Health*, p. 1012, *1917*, p. 212; Newark, Department of Health, *Monthly Bulletin*, N.S., Vol. I, No. 7 (July 1917); Bureau of Municipal Research, N.Y., "Survey," pp. 278-80.

83. *Newark Annual Reports, 1915, Board of Health*, p. 1012, *1917*, p. 212; Newark, Department of Health, *Monthly Bulletin*, N.S., Vol. I, No. 7 (July 1917); Bureau of Municipal Research, N.Y., "Survey," pp. 278-80.

8

Infant Mortality

The campaign to improve municipal milk supplies was part of a larger movement to save infant lives. If the infant mortality rate is any indicator, life in nineteenth-century America was not highly valued. During the 1880s and 1890s two out of every ten infants died before their first birthday. Infant deaths were the largest element in the mortality statistics, accounting for about 20 percent of the total number of fatalities in American cities.[1]

More than half of all infant deaths were preventable, the "results of poverty, ignorance, and neglect." The chief specific causes of infant mortality were: use of dirty, unwholesome, and bacteria-laden milk; improper feeding and maternal care; lack of prenatal care; unskillful assistance at delivery; and conditions associated with tenement living—overcrowding, dirt, poor ventilation, etc.[2]

Because it reflects the pull of a wide spectrum of social conditions, the infant mortality rate is a sensitive barometer of community health. As safe housing, medical care, education, and good nutrition become more generally available in a society, the infant mortality rate declines. A wealthy nation with a high infant mortality rate may be judged delinquent in using its resources to best advantage in protecting the public health. Then as now, the American infant mortality rate was scandalously high.

Until about 1900 or 1910 gastrointestinal disorders were the leading cause of death among infants. Because of difficulty in digestion and the rapid growth of bacteria in milk, the summer was the weeding-out time of infants. Every undertaker had a white hearse for infants and children. In the summer a steady stream of white hearses could be seen on the way to cemeteries. The exact cause of death was seldom known. In the loose medical terminology of the period, death was usually attributed to "cholera infantum," "summer complaint," or some other descriptive but nonmedical ailment indicating the presence of diarrhea.

TABLE 4

CAUSES OF INFANT MORTALITY IN NEWARK - 1902-1910

(PER 1,000 BIRTHS)

	Mortality from Respiratory Ailments	Mortality - Gastro Intestinal Disorders	Mortality - Congenital Debility	Mortality - Other Causes	Total
Avg. 1902 05	26.4	36.5	41.4	48.3	152.6
Avg. 1906 10	23.1	40.6	39.6	37.3	140.6

SOURCE: Julius Levy, Special Report of the Work Carried on by the Public Welfare Committee of Essex County for the Reduction of Infant Mortality in Newark, together with a Study of the Problem in Essex County and a Program for the City of Newark   (n.p.: Public Welfare Committee of Essex County, 1912), p.22.

Congenital malformations, birth injuries, premature birth, congenital debility, and other diseases peculiar to early infancy ran a close second to enteric disorders and have since surpassed them. Diseases of the respiratory tract, principally pneumonia and bronchitis, accounted for better than half as many deaths, and acute contagious diseases and all other ailments the rest.[3]

Around the turn of the century milk depots were established in tenement districts to provide safe, wholesome milk for the children of the poor. Bottles of milk were distributed free or for half price according to need. With the bottles came instructions printed in several languages on the keeping of milk and the care of infants in hot weather.

Before long it became apparent to reformers that clean milk constituted only one element and, at that, a secondary one, in saving infant lives. The major emphasis in child health work needed to be placed on teaching mothers to care for their babies. The task was not a simple one. While pamphlets on infant care could be given to middle- and upper-class women with good effect, the education of tenement mothers required a further effort. Burdened with the care of large families or with the need to work to supplement the family income, tenement mothers had neither the time nor the energy to study the child health brochures distributed by the board of health. Reaching these women called for a personal touch. It necessitated individual instruction provided for by visiting home nurses and by medical attendants at child health clinics.

In Newark the problem was shrouded by a veil of official apathy. In 1894 a pamphlet on infant health was written by Coit for the board of health. The pamphlet stressed the importance of good care and mother's milk or, if not available, of properly modified cow's milk, and contained instructions on the early recognition of illness, the handling of milk, and the nursing, feeding, clothing, weaning, and general management of infants. Parents were encouraged to pasteurize milk but were cautioned against the danger of sterilization by boiling.[4] That, however, remained the extent of the board of health's effort in this field for nearly twenty years. What little was done in Newark during this period to reduce the frightful toll of infant fatalities was the work of one man, Newark's milk crusader, Henry L. Coit.

Distressed by the needless loss of life, the widespread ignorance among the poor of infant hygiene, and the lack of suitable facilities for treating infants in the city's hospitals, Coit sought for eight years following his infant son's death to build a hospital devoted exclusively to the care of infants. Enlisting the support of prominent businessmen and physicians, Coit in 1896 founded Newark Babies Hospital (Coit Memorial Hospital), the second institution of its kind in the United States.[5]

The hospital was established with four purposes in mind: 1) to provide treatment for sick infants whose parents could not afford private medical care; 2) to train women to be intelligent caretakers of upper-class children; 3) to make safe, nourishing milk available to nursing indigent mothers; and 4) to afford physicians an opportunity to study at first hand the diseases of infancy.[6] The hospital admitted patients up to three years of age with acute noncontagious and enteric and respiratory disorders. A small amount of surgery was performed as well. The hospital had a capacity of about thirty-five beds, and was financed largely through private subscription and donation.[7]

A school was started to train nurses in infant care, also the second of its type in the United States, and clincs were established to treat minor infant ailments.[8] Certified milk was used, naturally, but owning to fears the poor would not be able to chill it, the milk was pasteurized.[9] With the bottles came instructions printed in English, German, Italian, and Hebrew.[10] During the first nine years an average of 160,000 bottles was distributed annually. About 250,000 bottles were dispensed yearly between 1907 and 1917, enough milk to feed about 400 to 600 babies.[11] The mortality rate for infants weaned on dispensary milk was between 2.7 and 6 percent, substantially below the city figure.[12]

Impressed by the dispensary's success and desirous of making infant care more readily available to the poor, representatives of the Bureau of Associated Charities, the Visiting Nurse Association, and the Newark Social Settlement met in 1908 and organized the Joint Committee on the Better Care and Feeding of Infants. With the aid and supervision of the medical department of Babies Hospital, four Baby Keep-Well stations were opened.[13] Mothers were encouraged to bring in their healthy infants for periodic checkups and consultations, milk was dispensed, and two nurses were employed to make follow-up home visits.[14]

Because of financial difficulties, in 1909 the expenses of the committee, except for the salaries of the nurses, were assumed by Babies Hospital, and in 1911 the committee was disbanded. The consultation centers were maintained, but the need to retrench compelled the hospital to eliminate the milk work of the stations and to dismiss one of the nurses.[15]

While Newark sat on its hands, other cities forged boldly ahead. In 1897 the first municipal milk depot was established in Rochester; by 1910 there were milk stations in forty-three cities. About the same time, by converting its milk depots into infant welfare centers, the New York City Health Department began providing a comprehensive program of health services for its burgeoning immigrant clientele.[16]

In a series of articles and editorials during the spring of 1911 the *Newark Evening News* described what other cities had achieved in protecting the health of infants and called upon the board of health to institute similar reforms.[17] The *News* reported that in Rochester the infant mortality rate for the summer months had been reduced more than 50 percent. "The Newark infant death rate," commented the *News*, "is neither natural, necessary, nor slight. They [the infant mortality figures of Rochester] show it to be abnormal, preventable, and criminal."[18]

In 1911 the Public Welfare Committee of Essex County commissioned Dr. Julius Levy, a Newark physician who had been active in infant and child-health conservation movements,[19] to examine the county's infant mortality.[20] Levy was authorized to undertake a test project and was charged with formulating a program for Newark which would "remove the infant mortality problem from private charity and philanthropy, and place it on a permanent and efficient basis."[21]

Levy believed the key to reducing infant mortality lay in inducing mothers to breast-feed their offspring and in employing visiting nurses to instruct new mothers in infant care. Coit, on the other hand, placed primary emphasis on improving the milk supply.[22] Furthermore, Levy argued that infant welfare work was the rightful province of the state, rather than of milk charities, such as had been established by Coit and Straus.

Four infant consultation centers were established, each staffed by a nurse assistant who visited new and expectant mothers in their homes. The nurses provided the women with elementary instructions in child care. Mothers were told how to dress their infants in warm weather, what to do about diarrhea, how to prevent rickets, and how to treat minor ailments. Because of the high incidence of deaths during the first months of life, a special effort was made to see mothers as soon after birth as possible.

With the cooperation of the Newark Board of Health, a good quality milk was made available through drugstores and home deliveries. The

mortality for the 509 babies who took part in the experiment was 2.3 perce
as contrasted with a mortality among infants of the same mothers born prio
to the opening of the stations of 13.9 percent.[23] "If we believe that the
most valuable asset of the community is the health and character of its
youth," commented Levy, "we cannot longer question the urgency of
making the conservation of infant life a special function of . . . a department of Child Hygiene."[24]

The failure of the board of health to implement the reforms recommended by Levy came under sharp attack in the report of the Russell Sage
Foundation. The report commented that of the over 1,300 infants who
died before their first birthday in 1910, "very possibly a fourth . . . and
possibly as many as a half of them, might have been saved by proper
preventive measures." "Several hundred preventable deaths in one year,"
the report continued, "is nothing short of a profound tragedy and cannot
much longer be regarded with indifference."[25]

Late in 1913 a division of child hygiene was established within the
health department on a trial basis. Julius Levy was appointed director of
the division, which was given $16,000 to prove its worth. The division's
limited funds confined its activities during its first year of operation (1914)
to two wards. The first and third wards were chosen, the wards with the
highest number of births and deaths and "the greatest degree of ignorance
and poverty." The first ward was populated by persons of Italian ancestry,
the third ward by Russian and Austrian immigrants.

Many persons, and perhaps most physicians, expected the experiment
to fail. "You can't teach these foreigners anything" was a commonly voice
sentiment among doctors. Moreover, at a time when standard pediatric
practice was curative rather than preventive, Levy was proposing to teach
"dumb" immigrants how to guard their newborn infants against serious
illness.

To establish contact with the young mothers in the area, consultation
centers were started in the public schools and nurses were sent into the
homes of every baby who had been delivered by a midwife or born in a
hospital. At the time hospitals were regarded as charitable institutions and
no self-respecting woman would give birth in one. In 1913 only 10 percent
of Newark births were in hospitals.[26]

The staffs at the centers were chosen for their motivation, adaptability,
and fluency in foreign languages. In keeping with contemporary pediatric
practice, great stress was laid on breast feeding (probably wisely, if for no
other reason than the difficulty of securing a high grade commercial milk).

The mortality rate for the babies supervised by the division was 1.1 percent, compared with a city-wide rate of 9.8 percent.[27]

In 1915 the appropriation of the division was increased to $10,000, enabling the division to extend its work to two more wards. Moreover, the president of the board of health announced that henceforth the well-being of infants would be given top priority.[28] Having established the division on a firm basis, Levy now began to effect a progressive and far-reaching program touching all phases of infant welfare work from prenatal care to the time the child entered school.

One of the first steps taken by Levy was to set in motion a plan for regulating and supervising midwives. Among Eastern European immigrant groups midwifery was an old and honored calling. Of the 11,107 babies born in Newark in 1914, 5,471 were ushered in by midwives.[29] (The author's father was delivered by a midwife some sixty-five years ago.)

Though the maternal and infant mortality rates for cases handled by midwives were sometimes lower than for those attended by physicians and hospitals, the conduct of midwives still left much to be desired. Of the 99 midwives practicing in Newark, 17 lacked the required state license; 50 failed to register births or did so late; 20 had no knowledge of silver nitrate; 9 carried drugs which the law forbade them to use, such as arsenic and strychnine; 16 had in their possession hypodermic syringes, uterine forceps, hard rubber catheters, specula, and other illegal instruments; 57 were considered unsanitary in person, home, or work; 70 did not consult physicians when confronted with complications; and 13 were suspected of being abortionists. Many medical authorities regarded midwifery as "a relic of barbarism" and hoped to have it legislated out of existence.[30]

Levy took the position that the majority of midwives were "willing, careful, and desirous of conforming to the law, and of rendering good service to their patients."[31] To prove that midwifery could be made respectable, Levy initiated a policy in which aid, education, and coercion were subtly intertwined. Midwives were required to register with the board of health and to attend board conferences and lectures on infant care. The state law regulating the licensing and work of midwives was strictly enforced, with the exception that practicing midwives who lacked the state educational requirements were allowed to take qualifying examinations in their lieu. Gradually the mistrust of midwives diminished to the point where they began asking the assistance of physicians in difficult pregnancies. In 1917 the board of health noted a major improvement in the quality of medical care offered by midwives.[32]

Levy was also anxious to reduce the large number of deaths from congenital debility in the first hours and days of life. To this end, prenatal clinics were established in the city's tenement districts, and an obstetrical outpatient department was opened at the city hospital.[33]

Besides reducing infant mortality, prenatal care also lessened the risk to new mothers. While the overall city-wide puerperal fever death rate in 1917 was 2.36 per 1,000 births, among women who had received prenatal care it was only 1.87.[34]

The work of the division was hampered by the city's antiquated method of collecting vital statistics. Births, marriages, and deaths were first reported to the city clerk who, in turn, furnished the board of health with transcripts. Because of the delay involved in securing these records, babies often did not come under the department's supervision for more than two weeks after their delivery. In 1915 no reduction occurred in the mortality rate of infants under one month. Though the necessity of double entries also entailed needless expense, the board of health was unable to obtain sole responsibility for the reporting of vital statistics. Levy, however, did secure better enforcement of a statute compelling the registration of births within five days after delivery. (The filing of death certificates, because they were needed for burials, required no special effort.) In 1914 unreported births, as discovered from death certificates, constituted 15 percent of all births; in 1916, just 9 percent.[35]

An all-out war was waged on gonorrheal ophthalmia, the commonest and most serious form of ophthalmia neonatorum (blindness in newborn infants), which in 1913 accounted for about 10 percent of all blindness in the United States. In 1881 Dr. Karl Sigmund Franz Crede, professor of obstetrics and gynecology at the University of Leipzig, Germany, and director of the Leipzig Lying-in Hospital, discovered that application of a silver nitrate solution to the eyes of newborn infants offered protection against the transmission of gonorrhea from infected mothers during childbirth. Since the drug also helped ward off other eye ailments, Crede proposed that it be applied to the eyes of all newborn infants. But there were many benighted persons who thought the use of silver nitrate was a slander on women's character. And for several decades "ignorance, carelessness, and prudery on the part of doctors, midwives, and the public held back the universal use of Crede's method."[36] Levy fought hard to dispel this prejudice and with the help of midwives and visiting nurses succeeded in reducing the number of cases of ophthalmia neonatorum by 40 percent in just two years. Meanwhile, measures were also instituted for the prevention, detection, and treatment of hereditary syphilis.[37]

Levy was also concerned about the care infants received in day nurseries and boardinghouses. In 1914 the board of health reported there were about 300 "destitute women" engaged in the boarding out of infants. Initially, Levy wanted to place foundlings whose mothers could not care for them in private homes. Subsequently, he proposed to establish a home for unmarried mothers where the mother could be rehabilitated without separating her from her child. Unfortunately, neither of these advanced proposals was acted upon prior to 1918. However, the division did gain the right to license boarding-out institutions (other than incorporated placing-out societies and institutions run by state agencies) and to regulate day nurseries.[38] The division also began the supervision and medical inspection of wet nurses. A wet nurse directory was compiled, and a system was arranged whereby physicians could obtain pumped breast milk or wet nurses for their patients, with special provision made for the indigent.[39]

Finally, Levy sought to promote the gospel of child health reform through the printed word and the schools. In 1914 26,000 leaflets were distributed by the division, and in 1917 600,000 copies of an exhibit on the proper care and feeding of infants were given away by the Prudential Insurance Company. "Little Mothers Leagues" were established in schools to instruct young girls in aiding their mothers and to prepare them for the day when they would have their own progeny to look after. Lectures and films were provided in schools and to social workers, women's clubs, and other groups concerned with the welfare of mothers and children.[40]

By 1919 the staff of the division had grown to include Levy, four physicians who worked in the clinics on a part-time basis, twelve nurses, and two clerks. Newark's infant mortality rate for the first six months of 1919 was the lowest of any city of its class in the United States.[41] The work of the division, wrote one informed source at this time, is "based on the most modern and progressive ideas of child hygiene work," and constitutes "an object lesson for other cities as well as for other divisions of the Newark Department of Health."[42]

In 1918 Levy became consultant to the recently established New Jersey State Bureau of Child Hygiene, where he again demonstrated the initiative and skill so manifest in his tenure as first director of the Division of Child Hygiene of the Newark Department of Health. For the next thirty years Levy divided his time between city and state work, helping to make Newark and New Jersey leaders in infant and child conservation.[43]

PLATE IV

NEWARK'S INFANT MORTALITY RATES, 1900—1922

Deaths under one year of age per 1,000 living births

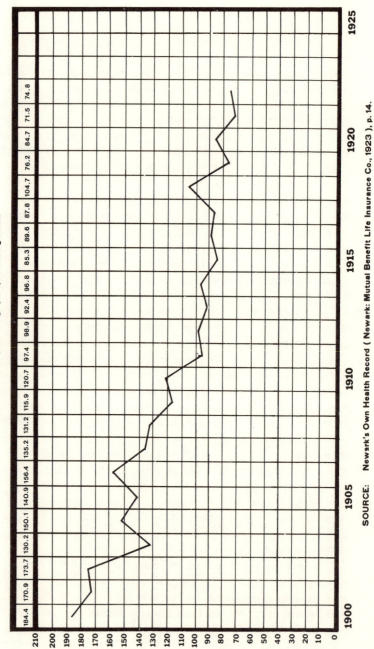

SOURCE: Newark's Own Health Record (Newark: Mutual Benefit Life Insurance Co., 1923), p. 14.

NOTES

1. Below, Appendix.

2. *Annual Report of Babies Hospital of the City of Newark for 1897-1898*, p. 23 (hereinafter referred to as *AR Babies Hospital*).

3. Milton J. Rosenau, *Preventive Medicine and Hygiene* (5th ed.; New York: D. Appleton and Co., 1913), p. 508, 6th ed., pp. 605-9.

4. [Henry Leber] Coit, *The Care of the Baby* (Newark: Medical Department of the Babies Hospital, Newark, N.J., 1894), p. 3.

5. Henry L. Coit, "Historical Sketch of the Babies Hospital," January 1914, Coit MSS., Box 13; letter, H. L. Coit to Dr. Hedges, n.d., Coit MSS., Box 1. Dr. Charles J. Kipp, founder of the Newark Eye and Ear Infirmary and one of Newark's best-known physicians, was a prime mover in the hospital's establishment.

6. *AR Babies Hospital, 1900*, p. 13.

7. A. W. MacDougall, *The Philanthropies of Newark: A Descriptive Directory* (n.p., 1916), p. 28; *AR Babies Hospital, 1908*, p. 28; letter, H. L. Coit to Dr. Hedges, n.d., Coit MSS., Box 1; Coit, "Historical Sketch of the Babies Hospital," pp. 10-11, Coit MSS., Box 13.

8. *Newark Evening News*, July 12, 1899.

9. *AAMMC Proceedings, 1910*, pp. 103, 116; *AR Babies Hospital, 1900*, p. 12.

10. *Newark Evening News*, July 12, 1899; Coit, The Medical Report of the Babies Hospital, Newark, N.J., to May 1, 1899, Coit MSS., Box 13.

11. *AR Babies Hospital, 1908*, pp. 46-47; *AAMMC Proceedings, 1910*, pp. 110, 113; *The Hospital Herald: Periodical of the Babies Hospital, Newark, N.J.*, XX, No. 2 (April 15, 1917), 10-11.

12. *AAMMC Proceedings, 1907*, p. 260, *1910*, p. 122.

13. Letter, H. L. Coit to Mrs. George E. Halsey, Sept. 30, 1910, Coit MSS., Box 4; A R Babies Hospital, 1909, p. 43.

14. Joint Committee on the Better Care and Feeding of Babies, *The Campaign in Newark to Lessen Infant Mortality* (n.p., 1908).

15. Letters, H. L. Coit to Mrs. George E. Halsey, Sept. 30, 1910, March 25, 1912, Coit MSS., Box 4.

16. Charles E. North, "Milk," *A Half Century of Public Health: Jubilee Historical Volume of the American Public Health Association*, ed. Mazÿck Porcher Ravenel (New York: American Public Health Association, 1921), p. 151; Philip Van Ingen, "The History of Child Welfare Work in the United States," *A Half Century of Public Health*, ed. Ravenel, pp. 306-8.

17. *Newark Evening News*, March 21, 22, 25, April 14, June 4, 1911.

18. Ibid., April 14, 1911.

19. Ibid., Feb. 23, 1911.

20. Julius Levy, *Special Report of the Work Carried on by the Public Welfare Committee of Essex County for the Reduction of Infant Mortality in Newark, together with a Study of the Problem for the City of Newark* (n.p.: Public Welfare Committee of Essex County, 1912), pp. 3, 8.

21. Ibid., p. 8.

22. Contrast Levy, *Special Report*, pp. 8-9, 24 with Coit, "Medical Milk Charities," *AAMMC Proceedings, 1910*, pp. 76-77, 79.

23. Levy, *Special Report*, pp. 14-15.

24. Ibid., p. 12.

25. *Newark Evening News*, June 5, 1913.

26. Thomas Neville Bonner, *The Kansas Doctor: A Century of Pioneerin 1850-1950* (Lawrence, Kansas: University of Kansas Press, 1959), p. 90; *Newark Evening News*, May 18, 1939.

27. *Newark Annual Reports, 1914, Board of Health*, pp. 708, 721.

28. *Newark Evening News*, Feb. 17, 1915.

29. *Newark Annual Reports, 1914, Board of Health*, pp. 704-32.

30. Ibid.; David L. Cowen, *Medicine and Health in New Jersey: A History*, Vol. XVI of *The New Jersey Historical Series*, eds. Richard M. Huber and Wheaton J. Lane (Princeton, N.J.: D. Van Nostrand Co., Inc., 1964), p. 172.

31. *Newark Annual Reports, 1914, Board of Health*, pp. 721-2; Julius Levy, *The Maternal and Infant Mortality Midwifery Practice in Newark, N.J.* (New York: William Wood & Co., 1918), p. 2.

32. *Newark Annual Reports, 1915, Board of Health*, pp. 1156-60, *1917*, pp. 292-4; N.J., *Public Health News*, I, No. 12 (July 1916), 288-9; IV, No. 2 (Jan. 1919), 9, Nos. 4-5 (March-April, 1919), 116-9; Newark, Department of Public Health, *Weekly Bulletin*, N.S., II, No. 6 (Feb. 5-12, 1916).

33. Ibid., *1914, Board of Health*, pp. 719-21; Julius Levy, *An Effective Child Hygiene Program: How Newark, N.J. Came to be a Leader in Infant Welfare Work* (New York: The Civic Press, n.d.), p. 4.

34. *Newark Annual Reports, 1914, Board of Health*, pp. 730-1, *1916*, pp. 1140-1.

35. *Newark Annual Reports, 1917, Board of Health*, p. 284.

36. Harry Wain, *A History of Preventive Medicine* (Springfield, Illinois: Charles C. Thomas, 1970), pp. 348-9; Rosenau, *Preventive Medicine*, 1st ed., pp. 60-62.

37. *Newark Annual Reports, 1915, Board of Health*, pp. 1961-2, *1916*, pp. 1371-2.

38. Levy, *Report on the Work of the Public Welfare Committee*, pp. 28-31; *Newark Annual Reports, 1914, Board of Health*, pp. 724-5, *1915*, pp. 1160-1.

39. *Newark Annual Reports, 1915, Board of Health*, p. 1154; Newark, Department of Health, *Weekly Bulletin*, N.S., Vol. I, No. 20 (Oct. 23-30, 1915).

40. *Newark Annual Reports, 1914, Board of Health*, pp. 718-19, *1915*, pp. 148-9.

41. Bureau of Municipal Research, N.Y., "Survey," pp. 242-6.

42. Ibid., p. 242.

43. Cowen, *Medicine and Health in New Jersey*, pp. 171-2; *Newark Evening News*, Jan. 27, 1969.

9

Tuberculosis

Over the centuries and throughout the world tuberculosis has stalked
man.[1] Pottery vases and other objects of art depicting the hunchback
condition associated with tuberculosis of the spine indicate tuberculosis
was no stranger to prehistoric man, a diagnosis confirmed by the indel-
ible imprint of the disease in prehistoric skeletons. Today, in America,
the disease can be found in places as disparate as an Indian reservation,
an Appalachian coal town, and an inner-city slum. Prior to 1918 tuberculosis caused more chronic disability and death than all other highly
acute contagious diseases combined.[2]

The social costs of tuberculosis were greater than for most other communicable diseases, since tuberculosis usually struck during the most
productive years of life. In 1900 tuberculosis accounted for one-third
of all deaths in the United States between the ages of fifteen and fifty-
four.[3] Hundreds of millions of dollars were spent annually in treating
and controlling the disease, to say nothing of the loss of productive labor to the economy. Yet the financial loss was as nothing when set
against the incalculable cost to society of disrupted family life brought
about by the separation, incapacitation, or death of a young parent.

The etiology of tuberculosis is fairly complex. A chronic infectious
disease of the lungs, the disease is primarily transmitted through droplet
spread.[4] Tubercle bacilli are expelled into the air in the acts of coughing,
sneezing, and expectoration. The microorganisms thus liberated may be
directly inhaled, as most often happens, or may stay suspended in the
air in droplet nuclei, frequently for long periods of time if the air is enclosed, until inhaled. The disease may also be communicated through
the inhalation of dust particles to which tubercle bacilli have adhered, or
through the mouthing of hands, food, utensils, and other objects recently contaminated with bacilli-laden respiratory secretions. The ingestion

of meat and milk obtained from diseased cows provides still another avenue of infection.

The course of clinical pulmonary tuberculosis is highly variable, ranging in severity from minor lesions that remain localized and are seldom discovered, to virtual destruction of the lungs and death. The path taken depends on several factors, such as the number and virulence of the invading microorganisms and the ability of the host to resist infection. The principal symptoms of a fully developed case of pulmonary tuberculosis are fever, loss of weight, breathlessness, pain in the side or shoulder, coughing, and blood spitting. In the nineteenth century, before there was effective therapy, the disease seemed to consume its feverish, shrunken victims and hence was called consumption.[5]

Ethnic groups displayed a varied susceptibility to tuberculosis. Immigrant groups were usually more seriously affected by the disease than native-born whites, and blacks continue to exhibit a very high vulnerability. Environmental factors, however, rather than genetic endowment, best explain these differences. Since fresh air, sunlight, rest, and nourishing food inhibit the disease's progress, the incidence of tuberculosis is closely tied to socioeconomic conditions. Thus war-ravaged nations in the first half of the twentieth century experienced sharp rises in their tuberculosis mortality rates after years of steady decline. Like infant mortality, tuberculosis is a weather vane of social conditions.[6]

At mid-century the death rate of tuberculosis in the United States was estimated at from 400 to 500 per 100,000 population. At that moment in history, with the industrial revolution well under way and exploitation of labor occurring on an unprecedented scale, tuberculosis confounded authorities on the disease by going into a nosedive. As a result of the enormous wealth produced by the industrial revolution—however unevenly divided among the population—the tuberculosis mortality rate by 1900 had dropped to 200 per 100,000 population.[7] The improved diet of the workingman and the free-standing suburban house of affluent commuters, to cite just a few of the period's improvements in living conditions, offered increased protection against the disease. It is also likely that the genetic out-breeding of persons with little resistance to the disease in conjunction with the enhanced immunity of the surviving population contributed to the waning of the pestilence.

Still, the American people could take little comfort in this windfall, for the disease continued to cause great suffering. During the first two decades of the twentieth century, tuberculosis killed about 160,000 persons annually in the United States. For every person who died from the disease there were nine persons with active cases and many more with inactive cases. Few persons escaped exposure to the disease, and as late as 1935 an estimated 60 to 90 percent of the adults living in American cities harbored the tubercle bacillus.[8]

Despite its annual ravages, tuberculosis went practically unnoticed before 1900. Tuberculosis lacks the characteristics best calculated to arouse fear. Individuals are not suddenly and violently bowled over. There are no dreaded symptoms,[9] and the disease does not cause paralysis, blindness, or disfigurement.

Of the 4,303 deaths which occurred in Newark in 1898, 611, or one-seventh of all, resulted from tuberculosis. Had smallpox, scarlet fever, diphtheria or any other contagious disease been responsible for the same mortality, the city would have proclaimed a quarantine against it, and the consequences would have been appalling. As the matter stands, however, the ravages of tuberculosis scarcely awaken comment except among those who have made it a specialty study, and by the great mass of people its slow, insidious but almost invariable fatal course is regarded as one of those evils which cannot be prevented.[10]

It was not until the discovery of the tubercle bacillus by Robert Koch in 1882 that any real attempt was made to combat the pestilence.[11]

Koch followed up his discovery of the tubercle bacillus with the announcement of tuberculin, a preparation made from the culture of the tubercle bacillus. Though tuberculin did not live up to its billing as a cure for tuberculosis, it did prove invaluable in detecting those susceptible to the disease when injected under the skin. A few years later another significant step was taken when it was discovered that tuberculosis could be diagnosed through bacterial examination of the sputum. Of even greater potential in diagnosing tuberculosis was Wilhelm Conrad Roentgen's discovery in 1895 of the X-ray.[12]

Somewhat before the time science began to come to grips with the disease, a method of treatment was found in the sanatorium. The sanatorium movement grew out of accumulated empirical folklore about the therapeutic value of fresh air, exercise, good diet, and rest. The use of a health regimen to treat tuberculosis was reinforced by the personal experiences of several prominent physicians, notably Edward L. Livingston Trudeau. In 1884 Trudeau founded the first sanatorium in the United States at Saranac Lake, New York.[13]

Sanatoriums did not provide the whole solution to the tuberculosis problem. As the number of patients seeking admission vastly exceeded the number of available beds, tuberculosis victims and their families and the public at large had to be educated in methods of home care and personal prophylaxis. A campaign of public education would constitute one of the outstanding attributes of the antituberculosis movement.

The loss of income and the disruption of family life brought on by the removal of a parent to a sanatorium posed grave social problems. At the same time, those who returned required new work suitable to their limited physical powers. But advertisements for "a light open-air job" usually went unanswered, and physicians despaired at sending patients back into the environment that had produced their sickness. Rehabilitation and medical social work were novel concepts in public health. A different kind of medical treatment joining the services of social-welfare agencies and allied health sciences was required. In the absence of government programs, voluntary agencies and charitable and civic organizations had to shoulder the burden of providing these new services. Thus tuberculosis could not be conquered by the medical profession and public health officials acting alone. Victory over tuberculosis would require a total marshaling of the community's resources.

In Newark the toll from tuberculosis was higher than in most American cities. Newark's average annual death rate from tuberculosis for the years 1901-1905 was 268.4 per 100,000 population, tenth highest in the nation among cities of over 100,000 population. Exceeding Newark in their death rates were five southern cities, where there were large Negro populations, Denver and Los Angeles, which attracted consumptives because of their sunny climates, and San Francisco and Cincinnati.[14]

The large number of deaths in Newark from tuberculosis was first noticed by the board of health in its annual report for 1886.[15] In 1894 tuberculosis was made a reportable disease, the disinfection of houses with tuberculosis was begun, and a circular, "Tuberculosis, Its Communicability and Prevention," was distributed.[16] Beginning in 1898 the bacteriological laboratory was employed against the disease, and the following year expectoration in public places was made illegal.[17]

The Newark Board of Health in 1903 completed a five-year epidemiological study indicating the environment in which tuberculosis was most likely to appear. The investigation revealed that indoor workers were

more prone to the disease than outdoor workers and that multiple cases
frequently occurred in blighted dwellings. About 20 percent of the victims either had tuberculosis in their families or had nursed cases.[18]

Mesmerized by the dizzying speed with which microbes were being
identified as the causes of acute, communicable diseases, medical men
sometimes let their enthusiasm cloud their judgment. At the turn of
the century the words "germ" and "disinfectant" had magical connotations.
Powerful throat swabs and gargles were employed indiscriminately
though the treatment was hazardous and of dubious value. Similarly,
pathogenic microorganisms were prematurely identified in cancer and
pellagra, and vaccines were announced that had not been adequately
tested.[19]

And so it was that in the early 1900s work was begun at the Newark
Board of Health on the development of a tuberculosis antitoxin. Two
antitoxins were developed which showed promise: 1) sepsis antitoxin,
which was prepared by immunizing horses to the pyrogenic bacteria
found in infected tissues and organs; and 2) tubercle antitoxin, which
was produced by immunizing horses to tubercle toxin. The first bottles of antitoxin were distributed in 1903 and the last in 1909, when the
practice was discontinued without comment.[20]

The board of health's other efforts to combat the pestilence were
equally futile. The antiexpectoration ordinance was not enforced,[21]
and physicians, unwilling to betray a patient's confidence, often hid the
disease.[22] Moreover, the board did little to alert the public to the menace of the white scourge.[23] Newark's death rate from tuberculosis in
1904 was an all-time high of 284.9 per 100,000 population.[24] The
Newark Evening News estimated the annual loss of earnings at $3 mil-
lion and asserted that the expense of burying the victims was more
than it would cost the city to mount an effective tuberculosis
drive.[25]

New Jersey trailed neighboring states in providing facilities for the
treatment of tuberculosis. As of 1905 the state had only eighteen sanatorium beds. After it was learned that tuberculosis was a communicable
disease, most general hospitals stopped admitting tuberculosis patients,
and the need for specialized institutional care became urgent. In the
years 1907-1910 a state sanatorium (Glen Gardiner Sanatorium) was established, and legislation was passed compelling the counties to establish
treatment centers.

In 1906 the New Jersey Association for the Prevention and Relief of

Tuberculosis was founded. The association concentrated its activities on education. Leaflets and pamphlets were distributed, stereopticon lectures were given, and graphic exhibits and displays were prepared. Visiting nurses were employed by the association to persuade persons afflicted with tuberculosis to enter sanatoriums or to attend clinics.[26]

The association was an effective lobbyist as well. As a result of the association's intercession, state legislation was enacted abolishing the public roller towel and the common drinking cup. Local public health authorities were authorized to remove dangerous cases of tuberculosis from the community. Moreover, an annual appropriation of $10,000 was secured for a continuing state educational campaign against the disease. Its objects secured and its work taken over by the state, the association in 1913 disbanded.[27]

The Newark Board of Trade, which had become alarmed about the economic cost of the disease, began sponsoring periodic exhibits[28] and along with other local organizations pressured the city to augment its tuberculosis programs. By this time a comprehensive plan for fighting tuberculosis had evolved and was in operation in parts of the United States and Europe. New York City's tuberculosis program, which ranked among the best, included the following requirements: 1) compulsory reporting and registration of all cases of pulmonary tuberculosis; 2) official supervision of isolation, especially of advanced cases; 3) free laboratory examination of all suspected cases; 4) education of the public; 5) disinfection; and 6) establishment of tuberculosis dispensaries and the use of home-visiting public health nurses.[29] Bowing to public pressure, the Newark Board of Health augmented its tuberculosis activities. In 1908 a more stringent tuberculosis reporting law was enacted.[30] In addition, a tuberculosis clinic was established at the city dispensary, and two nurses were assigned by the board of health to visit the homes of tuberculosis patients treated at the dispensary.[31]

In 1907 an appeal was made by two Montclair women in the name of indigent consumptives for the establishment of a municipal sanatorium in Newark. The appeal followed their discovery of an impoverished hatter who was dying of tuberculosis unattended in a cellar. Only the city hospital and St. Michael's then accepted tuberculosis patients. It was proposed to establish the sanatorium in the abandoned girls' cottage of the Newark City Home at Verona. The location of the home, on top of the second range of the Orange Mountains, was considered one of the best sites east of the Rocky Mountains for a sanatorium.

Residents of Verona, Montclair, and Caldwell tried to block the city's plans because of fears the sanatorium would impair property values and damage the future of their locale as a summer resort area. Their efforts failed, and in 1908 a sanatorium for incipient and moderately advanced cases was added to the city hospital, and in 1911 a county hospital, also for advanced cases, was established.[33]

The most important organization to enter the field against tuberculosis in Newark was the Committee of One Hundred, mainly comprising persons belonging to the Newark social register, which on April 1, 1909, reconstituted itself as the Newark Anti-Tuberculosis Association. The organization considered its purpose "educational rather than relief-giving" and hoped to pioneer new methods of combating the disease. Money for its activities was raised through contributions, benefit performances, and the sale of Christmas seals. The association distributed literature in eight languages. Posters and displays were placed in prominent store windows, exhibits were held in schools and libraries, and lectures were given wherever audiences could be gathered—churches, public playgrounds, nickelodeon theaters, factories, union halls, settlement houses, women's clubs, and fraternal and benevolent organizations.[34]

The association also functioned as a clearinghouse for the disposition of cases referred there by physicians and social service agencies. Specifically, it assisted victims of tuberculosis in obtaining relief and finding medical care. Tuberculosis patients were sent to clinics and aided in getting into sanatoriums. The indigent were put in touch with philanthropic organizations, and children who were orphaned or separated from their parents were placed in homes and institutions.[35]

A nurse was hired by the association to visit homes where there had been deaths from tuberculosis to be able to uncover at an early stage of the disease any secondary cases that might have occurred. In addition, the nurse did follow-up work on patients discharged from sanatoriums. Victims of the disease and their families were instructed in diet, cough control, sputum disposal, and care of personal articles and household furnishings. Whenever possible, sunny and well-ventilated rooms were set aside for the patient; in some instances, the porch was used as a bedroom.[36] Valuable assistance in this line of work was rendered by the Visiting Nurse Association of Newark.[37]

Through the efforts of Eleanor Aschenbach, a nurse who specialized in the care of tuberculosis patients, in 1908 an open-air treatment center was established. The center afforded daily observation and treatment for indigent patients who could not get into a sanatorium. Visitors at the camp received "The Cure," consisting of wholesome food, fresh air and sunlight, hygienic instruction, and medical supervision, the latter provided by physicians who donated their time. About thirty persons a day, mostly advanced cases, used the camp's facilities, including a few who were allowed to stay overnight. In 1909 the operation of the camp was taken over by the Committee of One Hundred, Miss Aschenbach staying on as supervisor and head nurse.[38]

At the request of the Newark Anti-Tuberculosis Association, which donated $1,000 toward the project, in the fall of 1910 an open-air school for pretubercular (anemic) children was started. The project was designed to care for children not yet suffering from active tuberculosis but who reacted positively to the tuberculin test. The school also admitted run-down children whose home environment was likely to expose them to the disease. Classes were conducted in an open-air pavilion, and students were fed nourishing meals. In the summer of 1911 the association converted its open-air treatment center into a summer school for children with tuberculosis, most of whom, since they were excluded from the public schools, did not receive an education. The experiment's success induced the board of education to transform its open-air school into a year-round center for tubercular students. The center accommodated some forty students, but, because of its location at the extreme southern end of the city, was poorly attended. Despite the pleas of the Supervisor of Medical Inspection of the Newark Board of Education, no new schools were started. Additional open air classes for anemic pupils, however, were established. By 1918, 12 schools had open-air facilities.[39] Unfortunately, the board of education and the board of health were frequently at odds, and the entire open-air school program no doubt suffered as a result.[40]

Partially as a health measure, philanthropic organizations endeavored to provide slum youths with a brief annual respite from their harsh environment. Every summer children from sweltering tenements were sent to the country for short vacations. Work of this kind was first undertaken in 1881 by the Female Charitable Society. It was supported with the aid of a small municipal appropriation and with the help of the *Newark Evening News*, which raised money through its annual Fresh Air Fund drive.[41]

The combined efforts of individuals, voluntary agencies, and public bodies notwithstanding, progress in the fight against tuberculosis was agonizingly slow. The average annual death rate for the years 1906-1910 was 258.2 per 100,000 population, or just about 4 percent lower than for the period 1901-1905. Evidence of real headway did not become apparent until the period 1910-1918, when the death rate fell to about 200 per 100,000 population.[42]

Dealing with tuberculosis presented formidable problems. For one thing, large numbers of cases went unreported. Fearing they would lose their jobs, many persons ignored early symptoms of the disease, choosing to delay treatment until the disease had become critical. It is likely that one-third of the cases of tuberculosis in Newark went undetected. The number of sanatorium beds barely kept pace with population growth. As of 1916 there were 200 beds available in Newark and Essex County. Estimating the minimum need at one bed for each death from tuberculosis, the board of health calculated that Newark was about 556 beds short.[43]

To add to the board of health's difficulties, a scandal was brewing at the municipal sanatorium in Verona. The sanatorium was a fire trap, records were ignored, and released patients received no follow-up care.[44] In the early part of 1915 the death rate at the sanatorium came under fire from the new president of the board of health.[45] Following a surprise visit to the hospital by the board in July 1915, the medical director and the superintendent and head nurse were dismissed when they were found absent without leave from their posts.[46]

The medical director, who had been charged with "incompetency and dereliction of duty," defended the results attained by the sanatorium and countercharged that the Board of Health had not made sufficient funds available to the institution. His defense had some merit, since the sanatorium had been opened woefully in need of repair[47] and "was never provided with adequate facilities to do the work for which it was intended."[48] At no time did its annual appropriation exceed $36,000, an amount barely adequate to feed and house the inmates of the sanatorium, but not great enough to expand its capacity or to make needed repairs.[49] The *Sunday Call* estimated that $250,000 was needed to rennovate the physical plant and that operating expenses would have to be quadrupled.[50]

In 1915 a division of tuberculosis was created within the department of health to administer the sanatorium.[51] Within two years the capacity of the sanatorium was nearly doubled.[52] Nevertheless, the city lacked the resources to run the institution effectively, and an earlier proposal to turn it over to the county, in whose hands it would be eligible for state funds, was revived. Negotiations were begun, and in August 1917—after interminable haggling over the value of the grounds—the transfer was completed.[53]

With the creation of a division of tuberculosis within the department of health, leadership in the tuberculosis movement passed from the private to the public sector of the community. As education of the public about the disease was already ongoing, the division concentrated on improving its field work. The nursing staff was more than doubled, and the number of clinics was increased from one to eight: four adult pulmonary clinics, two children's clinics, one laryngeal clinic, and one surgery clinic. At the clinics suspected cases were examined and a continuous check was made on persons returning from sanatoriums and on nonadvanced cases being treated at home. From mid-September through December 1915 the clinics were attended by 2,866 persons. In 1916 X-ray examinations for tuberculosis were begun.[54] To the shame of the city, in 1918 a clinic for colored citizens staffed by a Negro physician and a Negro nurse was established.

Not about to rest on its laurels, the division then proposed an ambitious tuberculosis program. Among the major recommendations called for were: open-air classes in every school, a preventorium for children exposed to tuberculosis, more clinics (and, in particular, a night clinic), additional nurses, day camps for tubercular children, a home for convalescents, and the exclusion of persons with tuberculosis from work in trades that brought them into direct personal contact with the public.[55] The latter was a matter of some importance. As of 1916 there were 206 food and drink handlers, 37 barbers, and 39 cigar makers in the city who were tubercular.[56]

One serious omission of the board of health was its failure to take note of cases of tuberculosis resulting from industrial hazards. "Since silicosis predisposes to tuberculosis, excessive inhalation of silica dust in such occupations as quarrying and foundry work [and in dusty trades such as felt and cigar manufacturing] should be avoided through proper sanitary and hygienic practices."[57] Newark's extensive industrial establishments rendered it acutely vulnerable. The absence of a division of industrial hygiene, probably in deference to the industrial leaders of Newark, constitutes a conspicuous failure of the department of health.[58]

As of 1918 the division of tuberculosis had precious little to show for its efforts. The death rate from tuberculosis for the first four years of the division's existence, 1915-1918, hovered at about 200 per 100,000 population.[59] But the breakthrough sought by the division was not far off. The division soon gained many of its objectives, and in 1919 the tuberculosis death rate started a steep decline. In 1922 Newark's tuberculosis fatality rate was only 99.1 per 100,000 persons, about 60 percent lower than when the tuberculosis campaign was launched around the turn of the century.[60]

In a survey of tuberculosis programs in effect in various cities in 1922, Newark was ranked as "approaching the perfect municipal tuberculosis unit."[61] But by 1920 public health authorities were nearing the limits of what they could hope to accomplish. Further significant advance in the battle against tuberculosis would await the development of new methods of diagnosis and treatment, such as mass X-ray screening of populations and chemotherapy.

NOTES

1. Joseph A. Bell, "Tuberculosis," Kenneth F. Maxcy and Milton J. Rosenau, *Preventive Medicine and Public Health,* ed. Philip E. Sartwell (9th ed., rev. and enl.; New York: Appleton-Century-Crofts, 1965), p. 210.

2. Henry Mitchell, "What Administrative Measures are Practicable for the Prevention of Pulmonary Tuberculosis?" *Trans. MSNJ, 1901,* p. 147; *Report of the Health Commission . . . 1874,* pp. 23-24.

3. Richard Harrison Shryock, *The National Tuberculosis Association, 1904-1954: A Study of the Voluntary Health Movement in the United States* (New York: The National Tuberculosis Association, 1957), pp. 62-63.

4. The following passages on the etiology, transmission, pathogenesis, and incidence of tuberculosis are based largely on Bell, "Tuberculosis," pp. 210-23.

5. Jean and René Dubos, *The White Plague: Tuberculosis, Man, and Society* (Boston: Little, Brown, 1952), pp. 4-6.

6. U.S. Bureau of the Census, *Eleventh Census of the United States, 1890: Report on Vital and Social Statistics,* II, 98; Dubos, *The White Plague,* pp. 140-1, 194-6.

7. Harry Wain, *A History of Preventive Medicine* (Springfield, Illinois: Charles C. Thomas, 1970), p. 338.

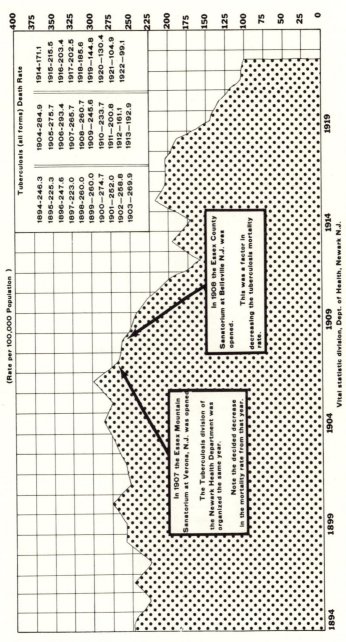

PLATE V

MORTALITY FROM TUBERCULOSIS, NEWARK, N. J.

(Rate per 100,000 Population)

Tuberculosis (all forms) Death Rate

1894—246.3	1904—284.9	1914-171.1
1895—225.3	1905—275.7	1915—215.5
1896—247.6	1906—293.4	1916—203.4
1897—223.0	1907—265.7	1917—202.5
1898—260.0	1908—260.7	1918—185.6
1899—260.0	1909—245.6	1919—144.8
1900—274.7	1910—233.7	1920—130.4
1901—252.0	1911—200.8	1921—104.9
1902—258.8	1912—161.1	1922—99.1
1903—269.9	1913—192.9	

In 1908 the Essex County Sanatorium at Belleville N.J. was opened.

This was a factor in decreasing the tuberculosis mortality rate.

In 1907 the Essex Mountain Sanatorium at Verona, N.J. was opened.

The Tuberculosis division of the Newark Health Department was organized the same year.

Note the decided decrease in the mortality rate from that year.

SOURCE: Newark's Own Health Record (Newark: Mutual Benefit Life Insurance Co., 1923), p. 11

Vital statistic division, Dept. of Health, Newark N.J.

8. Milton J. Rosenau, *Preventive Medicine and Hygiene* (6th ed.; New York: D. Appleton and Co., 1913), p. 43; *Newark Annual Reports, 1912, Board of Health*, pp. 161, 275.

9. Richard Harrison Shryock, "Medical History of the American People," *Medicine in America: Historical Essays* (Baltimore: The Johns Hopkins Press, 1966), p. 41; Shryock, *National Tuberculosis Association*, pp. 38-39.

10. *Newark Evening News*, June 7, 1900.

11. Dubos, *The White Plague*, pp. 58-59.

12. Wain, *A History of Preventive Medicine*, pp. 331-2; Shryock, *National Tuberculosis Association*, pp. 25-26.

13. Shryock, *National Tuberculosis Association*, pp. 28, 46.

14. U.S. Bureau of the Census, *Mortality Statistics, 1916*, pp. 42-43.

15. *Newark Annual Reports, 1886, Board of Health*, p. 564.

16. *Annual Report of the Board of Health, 1894*, p. 13.

17. *Newark Annual Reports, 1903, Board of Health*, pp. 1042, 1044; *Newark Sanitary Code . . . 1902, Addenda*, pp. 86-87.

18. *Newark Annual Reports, 1900, Board of Health*, pp. 50-53.

19. Shryock, *National Tuberculosis Association*, p. 27.

20. *Annual Report of the Board of Health, 1903*, pp. 52-55; *Newark Evening News*, Feb. 19, 1902, June 3, 1903.

21. *Newark Evening News,* April 4, 1901; *Yearbook of the Board of Trade, 1905*, p. 22.

22. *Newark Evening News*, Aug. 5, 1908.

23. *Annual Report of the Board of Health, 1898*, p. 27; *Newark Annual Reports, 1904, Board of Health*, pp. 959-60; *NJRCC*, V (1906), 91-93.

24. See Plate V.

25. *Newark Evening News*, Jan. 6, 1905.

26. Fred B. Rogers and A. Reasoner Sayre, *The Healing Art: A History of the Medical Society of New Jersey* (Trenton, N.J.: The Medical Society of New Jersey, 1966), pp. 182-3; David L. Cowen, *Medicine and Health in New Jersey: A History*, Vol. XVI of *The New Jersey Historical Series*, eds. Richard M. Huber and Wheaton J. Lane (Princeton, N.J.: D. Van Nostrand Co., Inc., 1964), p. 118; *Annual Report of the New Jersey Association for the Prevention and Relief of Tuberculosis for 1910-1911*, pp. 25-27 (hereinafter referred to as *ARNJTBA*).

27. Earnest D. Easton, "Forty Years of Progress in the Control of Tuberculosis," [N.J.] *Public Health News*, XXVII (December 1946), 180; *ARNJTBA, 1910-1911*, p. 5. *Minutes ECMS*, "Report of Committee on Tuberculosis," V, 96th Annual Meeting of the Essex County Medical Society, Feb. 17, 1915. The association was later reactivated and re-named the New Jersey Tuberculosis League.

28. *Yearbook of the Board of Trade, 1905*, p. 22, *1906*, pp. 19, 127 *1907*, p. 130.

29. Charles E. A. Winslow, *The Life of Hermann M. Biggs, Physician and Statesman of the Public Health* (Philadelphia: Lea and Febiger, 1929), pp. 132-4.

30. *Newark Evening News,* Aug. 5, 1908.

31. *Annual Report of the Newark Anti-Tuberculosis Association* (Committee of One Hundred) *for 1909-1910* (hereinafter referred to as *ARNTBA*).

32. *Newark Evening News,* Feb. 20-21, March 26, 1907; *Sunday Call,* March 24, 1907; *Newark Annual Reports, 1908, Board of Health,* pp. 353-4; *NJRCC,* VI (1907), 109-110, 150.

33. New Jersey Tuberculosis League, *Then and Now: New Jersey Tuberculosis League, 1906-1936* (n.p., n.d.), p. 10; *Minutes ECMS,* V, Feb. 17, 1915, "Report of Committee on Tuberculosis."

34. *ARNTBA, 1909-1910*, pp. 5-6, 10, 23, *1911-1912*, pp. 5, 7.

35. Ibid., *1909-1910*, p. 18, *1911-1912*, p. 5.

36. Ibid., *1909-1910*, pp. 14-18; *Neward Evening News*, January 27, 1905.

37. A. W. MacDougall, *The Philanthropies of Newark, New Jersey: A Descriptive Directory* (n.p., 1916), pp. 24-25; Rogers and Sayre, *The Healing Art,* p. 182.

38. Newark Public Library, N. J. Room, Vertical File, Newark, Public Health; *ARNTBA, 1909-1910,* pp. 19-22; MacDougall, *Philanthropies of Newark,* p. 36.

39. *ARNTBA, 1911-1912*, pp. 215-17, *1912-1913*, p. 12; *Newark Annual Reports, 1911, Board of Education*, pp. 215-17, *1912*, p. 96, *1918*, p. 201.

40. *Minutes ECMS,* V, Feb. 17, 1915, "Report of Committee on Tuberculosis."

41. *ARNTBA, 1911-1912*, pp. 13-15; *Newark Evening News,* June 3, 1905, June 4, 1909.

42. U.S. Bureau of the Census, *Mortality Statistics, 1916*, pp. 42-43.

43. *Newark Annual Reports, 1916, Board of Health,* pp. 1239-40; *1917,* pp. 161, 275; *NJRCC,* VII (1908), 184.

44. *Newark Evening News,* June 5, 1913, Dec. 12, 1914.

45. Ibid., Feb. 17, 1915; *Newark Annual Reports, 1914, Board of Health,* pp. 1087-9.

46. *Newark Evening News,* July 16, 1915.

47. *Newark Annual Reports, 1908, Board of Health,* pp. 353-4.

48. *Newark Evening News,* Feb. 24, 1917.

49. *Newark Annual Reports, 1908, Board of Health,* p. 353, *1909,* p. 310, *1910,* p. 551, *1915,* p. 1081.

50. *Sunday Call,* May 14, 1916.

51. *Newark Evening News,* July 16, 1915; *Newark Annual Reports, 1915, Board of Health,* p. 1073.

52. *Newark Annual Reports, 1917, Board of Health,* p. 271.

53. *Sunday Call,* May 14, 1916; *Newark Evening News,* May 20, 1912, July 14, 1916, Feb. 24, 1917; *Newark Annual Reports, 1917, Board of Health,* p. 271.

54. *Newark Annual Reports, 1915, Board of Health,* pp. 1088-91, *1916,* p. 1353.

55. *Newark Annual Reports, 1915, Board of Health,* p. 1091, *1916,* pp. 1354-6, *1917,* pp. 273-6, *1918,* pp. 308-16.

56. *Newark Annual Reports, 1916, Board of Health,* pp. 1355-6.

57. Bell, "Tuberculosis," p. 222.

58. Bureau of Municipal Research, New York, "Survey," pp. 258-59; Bell, "Tuberculosis," p. 222; *Newark Annual Reports, Board of Directors of the City Hospital, 1890,* p. 10.

59. See Plate V.

60. See *Newark Annual Reports, 1919,* pp. 333-40, *1920,* pp. 353-62, *1921,* pp. 381-92, *1923,* pp. 387-99.

61. *Newark Annual Reports, 1922, Board of Health,* p. 391.

10

Industrial Hygiene

From 1878 to 1883 the annual reports of the New Jersey Board of Health featured a series of articles on mortality in industrial trades with special focus on the hat industry. In an inspection of 25 factories in the Newark area employing nearly 1,600 operatives, hatters were found to be suffering from a high incidence of tuberculosis, rheumatism, and catarrhal inflammations. The reason, however, for the interest of physicians and reformers in the hat industry was the prevalence of the "shakes," muscular tremors induced by mercury poisoning, whence the expression "mad as a hatter." In the course of the investigation employees were observed inhaling volatilized mercury and fine fur fibers. Some men reported the expectoration of black dust one or two weeks after quitting work. Volatilized mercury did not provide the only risk. Many employees had to work in wet clothing or were subjected to sudden and drastic changes of temperature. Diseases of the respiratory tract, tuberculosis in particular, caused the greatest mortality. Of the 500 hatters who died in Newark and Orange in the years 1873-1882, 265, or 53 percent, died of tuberculosis. The life expectancy of a hatter was less than forty-one years.[1]

Medical interest in the risks peculiar to various kinds of employment dates back many centuries.[2] Hippocrates described the hazards faced by miners in ancient Greece. Bernadino Ramazzini, the great Italian physician, compiled a textbook on occupational diseases in 1700. But there was little public interest in industrial hygiene until the Industrial Revolution. The substitution of mechanical energy for human and animal power that began about 1800 witnessed a sharp escalation in violent work accidents. Exposure to a wide assortment of toxic substances was equally injurious to the worker's health.

Work conditions in factories were inhumane. Factories were designed to cram as many machines and workers into as small an area as possible

135

without thought to the risks involved. Working in a factory was akin to
running an obstacle course. Loose pulleys, projecting setscrews, and exposed saws and flywheels menaced the employee's life and limbs. Away
from his machine, the worker had to watch out for open hatchways and
hoistways. Plants provided almost no amenities for their employees and
seldom were equipped to handle emergencies. Fire escapes and overhead
sprinklers were frills found in only a few establishments. Restrooms
either did not exist or lacked adequate facilities. Workrooms were not
cleaned since it was popularly believed that a dirt-covered floor was a
sign of productivity. In all matters the protection of property took precedence over the conservation of human life.

The number of work-related maimings and deaths during the early
stages of industrialization was staggering. Workers were so much grist
for industry's satanic machines. Maimed and severed limbs made up the
scrapheap of the Industrial Revolution. "As a matter of fact, the chances
were better than even that the average worker would be killed, crippled,
or injured by an industrial accident in the course of his employment
life span."[3] In 1912 Metropolitan Life Insurance Company calculated
that the life expectancy of a twenty-year-old white male worker was 15
percent below the national average.

Lack of regard for the health and safety of workers can not be attributed solely to the callousness of entrepreneurs and plant managers.
Workers no less than businessmen believed that a certain amount of
hardship was unavoidable and was the price of progress. In addition, the
new machinery of the Industrial Revolution had to be used before the
parameters of industrial hygiene could be determined.

The first state to attempt to lessen the hazards of industrial employment was Massachusetts. In 1867 the Bay State began the appointment
of factory inspectors. A decade later legislation was enacted compelling
the installation of guardrails for dangerous machinery. But except for
Massachusetts, industrial hygiene did not exist in the United States
prior to 1900, though its value had already been shown in England and
on the continent.

Alabama tackled the problem of industrial hygiene in a rather different manner by making factory owners liable for accidents to their employees. The legislature thus hoped to provide employers with an incentive
for curbing the state's appalling industrial accident toll, which had added
greatly to local relief rolls. Similar laws were soon adopted in other
states, but their intent was not realized. Employers were able to pro-

tect themselves against liability suits by invoking any of three common law defenses. The doctrine of contributory negligence absolved the employer of liability if the employee was in any way responsible for the accident. Owners similarly escaped culpability if a co-worker was at fault. Lastly, under the "assumption of risk" interpretation of the courts, workers were refused compensation for accidents resulting from dangers held to be inherent in the occupation (on the reasoning that the worker was compensated for the risks and had knowingly agreed to them when he signed on). Even if these hurdles could be surmounted, employees seldom were able to recover sufficient damages to make a costly and time-consuming court fight worthwhile. Before the enactment of a workmen's compensation law in New Jersey, only one worker out of ten received compensation in cases of permanent disability, and 75 percent of his award was consumed in litigation.[4]

New Jersey's baptism in the field of labor relations occurred in 1878 with the establishment of a Bureau of Statistics of Labor and Industries. At a time when "industrial accidents and occupational diseases were among the problems conspicuously avoided by most labor bureaus,"[5] the New Jersey Bureau of Statistics of Labor and Industries used its fact-gathering powers to delineate the social costs of unbridled industrialization. In 1889 and irregularly thereafter the bureau devoted part of its annual report to the effect of labor on employees' health and trade life in several of New Jersey's principal industries. The reports of the bureau shed light on child labor, the health of working women, the insecurity of industrial employment, and other topics that subsequently became subjects of legislation.[6]

In 1885 a Bureau of Factory and Workshop Inspection was established to enforce a general factory act enacted that year. The amended statute stipulated an extension of a prior ban on child labor, the reporting of accidents, and the placing of safeguards on hatchways, elevators, and hazardous machinery. The bureau was also given supervision over the sanitary condition of factories and bakeshops. Handicapped by the numerous loopholes provided manufacturers and parents, the bureau failed abysmally in its main task, that of curtailing the exploitation of child labor;[7] many factory owners did not even permit inspectors to enter their plants.[8]

The period 1892-1904 witnessed a near halt in factory inspection. Organized labor and Progressives attributed the bureau's inactivity to the malfeasance of the chief inspector, John C. Ward, a farmer and former

state senator with a record of hostility toward labor. Governor Franklin
Murphy publicly censored Ward for neglect of duty and secured special
legislation to obtain his suspension. In 1904 the Bureau of Factory and
Workshop Inspection was succeeded by the Department of Labor, and
Lewis T. Bryant was appointed commissioner of labor.

The Department of Labor was organized in tandem with new factory
and child labor legislation. Children under fourteen were barred from
employment in workshops, factories, and mines, and children under sixteen were forbidden to work at jobs where there was exposure to certain
occupational diseases or the risk of physical mutilation. Enforcement
of child labor laws was facilitated through the enactment of more stringent compulsory education laws and amendments to extant child labor
legislation. The department's authority was extended to lighting and to
the protection of workers from vessels containing molten metal or liquid.
In certain instances, the department was empowered to require the installation of blowers to shield workers from dust. Finally, separate restrooms were required for male and female employees.[9]

For the next two decades the Department of Labor spearheaded the
drive for industrial hygiene reform. The annual reports of Commissioner
Lewis T. Bryant embodied much of what was best in Progressivism:
moral indignation, a pragmatic and scientific approach to social problems,
and faith in man and the democratic process. Writing in 1913, Bryant observed that both New Jersey and the nation had been slow to recognize
their responsibility for guarding workers against industrial diseases. Bryant
argued that far from saving money, the failure to protect workingmen
had resulted in a loss of productive labor and an increase in the number
of dependent widows and orphans.

> Economic questions aside, the State owes to workers who are, to a
> great degree, helpless to protect themselves, a constant humane policy
> of protection; which shall diminish those unnecessary accidents, in-
> dustrial deaths, and occupational diseases, which the experience of
> other countries has proven are a needless loss and sacrifice of child-
> hood, womanhood, and manhood to a false idea of social economy.[10]

Though a Republican, Bryant was kept in office during the Wilson governorship and every succeeding governorship until his death in 1923.
With Bryant at the helm, New Jersey became a leader in industrial
hygiene.[11]

The factory laws in force when the Department of Labor began its career were couched in broad, vague phrases. Thus the occupational disease law compelled employers to provide "reasonably effective devices, means and methods to prevent the contraction by . . . their employees of any illness or disease incident to the work or process in which they are engaged." Other safety ordinances required "proper" machine guards, "sufficient" ventilation, and "practical" fire control measures. The wide discretionary powers given factory inspectors by these vague phrases led to variances in enforcement from one area of the state to another. Furthermore, without the backing of a specific legislative mandate, inspectors were reluctant to arouse the wrath of industrialists. "Initially factory inspectors were about as welcome in many plants as a federal revenue agent was in the hills of some of the southeastern states."[12] Hence inspectors customarily limited their activities to rectifying only the most flagrant abuses.

There followed a relatively brief interval at the beginning of the twentieth century in which narrowly constructed and excessively detailed laws were enacted. Fortunately, the more comprehensive phraseology of earlier statutes was retained. The elasticity of these earlier laws combined with the wide latitude given the department to fashion administrative rules and regulations enabled the department to keep abreast of technological changes without having to seek new, hard-to-obtain legislation.[13]

Protection of workers against industrial diseases evolved more slowly than factory safety legislation. Maimings were electrifying, whereas sickness was pedestrian. Workers who were conscious of job accidents because of the anguish ensuing from the loss of a limb frequently ignored the insidious advance of tuberculosis, silicosis, and lead, mercury, and arsenic poisonings. In 1907 and 1908 the United States Bureau of Labor circulated monographs written by Dr. Frederick L. Hoffman, the chief statistician of Prudential Insurance Company, on consumption in the "dusty trades." By 1915 several insurance companies rated these trades as hazardous to health and either refused to write policies for high-risk employees or else made the premiums prohibitive.[14]

In 1911 the Department of Labor was given carte blanche power to compel the installation of exhaust fans or, in some other manner, to eliminate dust, noxious fumes, and excessive heat, moisture, and humidity from workrooms. The following year the department conducted an exhaustive inquiry into the health and safety of New Jersey workers. Eight matters of industrial hygiene were considered:

1. Exposure to some fifty industrial poisons, whose harmful effects may result from their fumes, gases, or solution.

2. Exposure to nonpoisonous but harmful dusts.

3. Exposure to bad air due to lack of space and imperfect ventilation.

4. Exposure to steam and dampness.

5. Exposure to excessive heat or cold, frequently in alternation.

6. Exposure to eyestrain due to glare or insufficient lighting.

7. Exposure to overspeeding, monotony of motion, overexertion, and excessive noise.

8. Exposure to occupational intemperance.

The department concluded:

1. That industrial poisonings, due especially to lead and mercury, were alarmingly frequent.

2. That such industrial poisonings could be prevented by sanitary methods in the industries affected.

3. That industrial tuberculosis was a serious evil in the so-called dusty trades and in all metal grinding, buffing, and polishing processes.

4. That proper mechanical exhaust ventilation and blower systems could effectively protect the worker against the once inevitable tuberculosis risks.

The Department of Labor then issued Sanitary and Engineering Industrial Standards. Meanwhile, a small but growing number of businessmen had come to accept the mutuality of interest of worker, employer, and government in reducing job-related sicknesses. Enlisting their aid, the department vigorously attacked the problem of sickness in industrial employment. In 1912 the department also required the reporting of occupational diseases, but the statute was poorly enforced.[15]

No discussion of the evolution of industrial hygiene in New Jersey would be complete without mention of the Employer's Liability (workmen's compensation) Act of 1911. The law compelled employers to pay the medical and hospital costs arising out of all work accidents plus 50 percent of the worker's wages for the period of his incapacitation. Compensation was originally limited to accidents, but by 1921 was extended to certain occupational maladies. The adoption of workmen's compensation provided a financial incentive for improving work conditions. Some of the insurance companies that wrote industrial policies undertook research in industrial hygiene. Inspectors sent out by the companies advised factory owners on safety and health installations. Desirous of reducing the cost of insurance premiums, businessmen began to pay closer attention to their employees' well-being on the job. The years 1911-1912, when the workmen's compensation movement came to its first fruition in the United States, mark a turning point in the history of American industrial hygiene.[16]

The pattern of industrial hygiene supervision that emerged in the United States placed primary responsibility in the hands of state agencies. Nevertheless, by the second decade of the twentieth century a few cities had come to realize the importance of inspecting food handlers for communicable diseases, of enforcing sanitation in the processing and sale of food, of regulating tenement sweatshops, and of assisting the state in the overseeing of local factory conditions. Because of Newark's concentration of industrial establishments, its citizens were particularly in need of protection.[17]

In 1919 the New York Bureau of Municipal Research charged the Newark Department of Health with having failed to discharge its obligations to the city's industrial workers.[18] Similarly, long after the state had become involved in abating slum housing, the department continued to ignore the hovels and sweatshops that abounded in Newark tenement districts. It is difficult to escape the conclusion that the department shirked its responsibilities in these areas so as not to antagonize Newark business leaders. It was the prevailing sentiment of the vocal elements in the city that it was "better that a few employees should be inhumanely treated than that an industry should leave town."[19] A small reform was made in 1920 when a division of industrial hygiene was established within the Newark Health Department to investigate cases of lead, mercury, and arsenic poisonings.[20]

NOTES

1. Leban Dennis, "Hatting as Affecting the Health of Operatives," *ARNJBH, 1878*, p. 69; Ezra M. Hunt, "The Hygiene of Occupations: General Introduction," *ARNJBH, 1883*, p. 158; J. W. Stickler, "The Hygiene of Occupations: Diseases of Hatters," *ARNJBH, 1883*, pp. 178, 182, 184-8.

2. The following remarks are based on Philip H. Burch, Jr., *Industrial Safety Legislation in New Jersey* (New Brunswick, N.J.: Bureau of

Government Research, Rutgers University, 1960), pp. 1-3; Philip Charles Newman, *The Labor Legislation of New Jersey* (Washington: American Council on Public Affairs, 1943), pp. 115-6.

3. Burch, *Industrial Safety Legislation*, p. 2.

4. Ludwig Teleky, *History of Factory and Mine Hygiene* (New York: Columbia University Press, 1948), pp. viii-xi; Burch, *Industrial Safety Legislation*, p. 3-4; Leo Troy, *Organized Labor in New Jersey* (Supplementary Volume, *The New Jersey Historical Series*, eds. Richard M. Huber and Wheaton J. Lane, Princeton, N.J.: D. Van Nostrand Co., Inc., 1964), p. 165; Monroe Berkowitz, *Workmen's Compensation: The New Jersey Experience* (New Brunswick: Rutgers University Press, 1960), p. 116.

5. Robert H. Bremner, *From the Depths: The Discovery of Poverty in the United States* (New York: New York University Press, 1956), pp. 74, 283.

6. Troy, *Organized Labor*, pp. 164-6; Newman, *Labor Legislation*, pp. 112-3; N. J., Bureau of Statistics of Labor and Industries, *Annual Report*, p. 23.

7. Since the protection of children was provided almost entirely through the general provision for the health and safety of factory workers, the evolution of child labor legislation has been largely omitted. For further information see Arthur Sargent Field, *The Child Labor Policy of New Jersey* (Cambridge, Mass.: American Economic Association, 1910).

8. N. J., Inspector of Workshops and Factories, *Annual Report, 1900*, pp. 11-12, 312-7; Newman, *Labor Legislation*, p. 113.

9. Newman, *Labor Legislation*, pp. 105, 114; Troy, *Organized Labor*, pp. 164-6.

10. N.J., Department of Labor, *Annual Report, 1913*, p. 4 (hereinafter referred to as *ARNJDL*).

11. Troy, *Organized Labor*, pp. 167-8.

12. Burch, *Industrial Safety Legislation*, p. 5.

13. Ibid., pp. 5-7.

14. George Martin Kober, "History of Industrial Hygiene and its Effects on Public Health," *A Half Century of Public Health: Jubilee Historical Volume of the American Public Health Association*, ed. Mazÿck Porcher Ravenel (New York: American Public Health Association, 1921), p. 397; *ARNJDL, 1915*, p. 50.

15. *ARNJDL, 1913*, pp. 6-8, *1914*, p. 22, *1915*, p. 21; New Jersey Sanitary Association, *Official Convention Number, Fifty-Second Annual Meeting* (1875-1926), p. 52.

16. Berkowitz, *Workmen's Compensation,* pp. 3-4; Burch, *Industrial Safety Legislation,* pp. 4-5; Newman, *Labor Legislation,* p. 108; Teleky, *History of Factory and Mine Hygiene,* pp. 73-74.

17. *ARNJDL, 1915,* pp. 21-26; *Newark Annual Reports, Board of Directors of the City Hospital, 1890,* p. 10.

18. Bureau of Municipal Research, N.Y. "Survey," p. 259.

19. Willard D. Price, *The Ironbound District: A Study of a District in Newark, N.J.* (Newark: The Neighborhood House, 1912), p. 25.

20. *Newark Annual Reports, Board of Health, 1920,* p. 261.

11

Tenement Housing

Law and tradition have sanctified the belief that a man's home is his castle. But for the poor of some fifty to one hundred years ago, home was a jerry-built structure in which large families were crowded together. Constructed without regard to health and safety, home was also a fever nest and a fire trap. Parenthetically, about the sole place where the workingman could find the relaxation his day's toil entitled him to was the neighborhood saloon. In testimony to the workingman's plight, the per capita consumption of alcohol in the United States nearly doubled in the last two decades of the nineteenth century.

The housing of the lower class improved only slightly during the nineteenth century. Initially, the sole building regulations in force pertained to structural matters and were intended to protect property. Enacted in an ad-hoc manner, they were subsequently rationalized in building codes. Plumbing regulations were added after the Civil War to guard against sewer gas, effecting an improvement in households fortunate enough to enjoy indoor plumbing. Progress in these areas was offset by the appearance of tenements in the older core sections of the nation's metropolises. Originally conceived of as multiple-dwelling units designed to provide cheap lodgings for the working class, tenements soon became synonymous with slum housing and urban blight.[1]

With the development of mass transit about 1880, the need of workers to reside within walking distance of their jobs ended, and vast tracts of low-cost land were opened for settlement. White-collar employees and skilled artisans flocked to the suburbs, where cheap vacant land made possible the construction of large houses equipped with the latest sanitary fixtures. The trolley thus released the middle class from the crowded tenements of the inner city. A new type of housing pattern and land use emerged. All along the suburban tracks of the trolley lines unbroken stretches of free-standing houses appeared, each house set back from the street by a lawn and separated from its neighbor by a narrow service alley. Though the rigid grid pattern of street design and the rectangular plot division employed by suburban developers, whatever the contour of the land, did not always measure up to the highest contemporary standards of land use, suburban houses were far superior to the slum rookeries of tenement districts. Unfortunately, those with small incomes remained trapped in the city in slum housing, while the suburbs underwent a rigid class segregation.[2]

Social reformers viewed the wretched housing of the urban poor primarily in terms of its pernicious effects on health and morals. Health surveys indicated a high incidence of consumption, typhus, and typhoid fever in basement dwellings. Concern about "vitiated" air (air saturated with carbon dioxide as a result of poor ventilation) touched off a spirited debate over the number of cubic feet of air space needed per adult or child indoors. The prudish strain in American society aroused an inordinate concern about the moral degeneracy of tenement dwellers. It was believed that congestion produced a morbid curiosity about sex among young persons and fostered illicit relationships among household residents. That slums bred prostitution and drunkenness was evident to all.[3]

Though by 1918 nearly every area of Newark was serviced by municipal water and sewerage, the laying of sewer and water mains did not insure the use of flush toilets or a water tap at the sink. The city's responsibility for providing sanitary services ended at the street line. A property owner could tap in at the curb, but it was at his own expense; also, he had to provide his own plumbing and fixtures. This division of responsibility worked to the satisfaction of a majority of city dwellers, but left the poor without adequate sanitary facilities. Affluent homeowners and builders for the middle-class market were willing to pay the small costs involved in obtaining the latest sanitary improvements. This was not true of tenement owners, who generally provided the least amount of services the law allowed. The Newark Board of Health was authorized to require property owners abutting on a sewer or a waterline to tap in, but the board was unwilling to prosecute politically influential landlords. Consequently, many problems of environmental sanitation that were under control in the larger community, such as water supply, disposal of wastes, and vector eradication, persisted in microcosm in tenement districts. Perhaps as many as one-third of urban dwellers were denied the rudimentary essentials of a safe, sanitary house because they were poor.[4]

Since filth is the handmaiden of disease, the city's failure to provide indoor sanitary facilities for the poor sustained a high incidence of morbidity in tenement districts. Over 80 percent of the deaths from consumption in Newark occurred among persons who lived in tenements. Gastrointestinal diseases were fostered by want of adequate bathroom facilities. Human fecal matter was carried on the feet of flies from privies and defective plumbing fixtures to exposed foods or to the nipples of milk bottles, thus causing infant diarrhea. Crowded apartments incubated respiratory disorders and acute infectious diseases. The extent of warped physical and mental development brought on by living in squalor and by lack of privacy can only be guessed.[5]

Until the twentieth century most Newarkers lived in one- and two-family wooden-frame houses.[6] In the 1890s tenement houses began to rise in the Ironbound and Hill sections. The first structure in Newark specifically designed as a tenement was a three-story building with two rental units on each floor. When hordes of immigrants began arriving about 1890, the buildings were divided and subdivided into as many as sixteen apartments. In addition, numerous one- and two-family houses were converted into tenements. By 1904 there were over 11,000 tenement houses in Newark. Other cities in New Jersey underwent similar transformations, and in 1904, three years after the passage of the pioneering New York Tenement Law of 1901, New Jersey enacted the nation's first state-wide tenement house law.[7]

The Board of Tenement House Supervision established under the 1904 law came into existence after a temporary tenement house commission had recommended "radical changes." The explosion in tenement house construction beginning about 1890 had caused conditions that "had to be seen to be comprehended."

Foul malodorous privy vaults, filled to the yard level and, in many cases, overflowing into the yards and draining into adjacent cellars; the floors and even the walls, covered with an accumulation of fecal matter; dark unventilated cellars, partially filled with garbage and refuse of all kinds and littered with heaps of discarded bedding, rags, paper and other inflammable material; broken soil and waste pipes discharging into the cellars; sleeping rooms so dark that even in broad daylight objects at a distance of only a few feet were indiscernible; broken and dilapidated stairs holding out menace to life and limb, and an almost total absence of means of escape in case of fire, were among the features of the problem.[8]

The commission assured the governor and the legislature it presented "simply the bare facts . . . without embellishment of any kind, and that the pictures of overcrowding, improper sanitary regulations . . . the squalor, the filth, the standing invitation to epidemics found in many places in the larger cities are not one whit overdrawn."[9] The principal needs uncovered by the commission were: light and ventilation, better sanitary arrangements, more adequate means of escape from fires, larger rooms, and more spacious apartments.

Borrowing the language of the New York Tenement Law of 1901 (and in accordance with the standard classification adopted by the United States Census in 1890), tenements were defined as dwellings containing three or more families.[10] Stringent specifications were established for the construction of new tenements. Among the more than 200 sections of the code which command attention are provisions for: a modern sanitary water closet in each apartment; access to direct outside light and air in each room; iron fire escapes in buildings of a certain size; a sink in every dwelling; and at least one room in each apartment with a minimum of 120 square feet of floor space and no room with less than 70 square feet. The law also provided, within certain limits, for the alteration of existing tenements. Tenements built before the law went into effect were required to have a water closet for every two families and a sink in each apartment, except where a sink had already been installed on each floor. Further improvements called for the installation of windows in dark rooms, fire escapes, and the cleaning and repairing of plumbing, sanitary appliances, stairs, roofs, ceilings, etc.[11]

There were four fairly distinct types of rental dwellings in Newark about the time the board began its work.[12] First there was the three-story wooden tenement containing one or two rental units on each floor. Speaking tubes running between the front porch and each apartment were a common feature, and a visitor having announced himself through the tube was admitted into a building by means of an electrical appliance controlled from the apartment to which he sought entrance. The apartments usually contained from four to six rooms and were fairly large. This type of house was mainly found in blocks containing three and six tenements.

Scattered blocks of tenements, usually four stories high and containing from eight to sixteen dwellings, were found in the older, downtown area. These were the dwellings of the less well-to-do among the working class. Running water was not provided and, in the absence of flush toilets, communal privies had to be used. A common type of apartment found in these buildings was known colloquially as a "railroad" flat. The four rooms extended all in a line from front to back. The windows in the parlor, or "sitting" room, overlooked the street. At the other end of the apartment, the kitchen window opened on the backyard. The intervening rooms were unlighted and airless save for what little breeze and sunshine filtered in from the outside rooms.

One- and two-family houses from the pre-Civil War era formed the third type of housing. Structurally they were similar to the superior type of two-family house described below, but lacked their spaciousness, attractiveness, and convenience. Bathrooms were rare and the rooms were generally small. With the making of a few modest renovations, most of the single-family cottages had been converted into two-family houses.

The fourth and best type of rental dwelling was the two-family house of modern construction. It was the accommodation of the professional and business class. Besides having the most modern sanitary amenities, including perhaps a tub, the apartments often were furnished with heat from a furnace in the basement. Commonly there were three attics, which were assigned by arrangement. The houses were of many different designs representing a wide range of rentals, but even the bottom rent was beyond the means of all but a few highly skilled artisans.

Despite the existence of tenements, housing was less congested in Newark than in the great ports along the Atlantic seaboard. Newark did not contain miles of attached row houses or blocks of more than one tenement crowded onto the same lot (as could be found in Philadelphia and New York, respectively). Because houses were not built back to back, few apartments stood in the shadow of large tenements or had but a single exposure onto a dark foul-smelling alley. With the exception of basement dwellings and the interior rooms of railroad flats, apartments in Newark usually received sunshine and fresh air.[13]

On the other hand, the census of 1890 revealed an occupancy rate in Newark of 7.81 persons to each dwelling; of 28 cities with populations of over 100,000 only 6 had higher rates. As was true of other American

communities, the supply of new housing in Newark simply did not keep
up with population growth, resulting in dangerous overcrowding. Already
large households had to expand to take in friends and relatives who were
unable to find lodgings because of the tight housing market. While families felt compelled to take in relations, boarders were taken in for the
rent they paid. The worst overcrowding occurred in cheap lodging houses,
where patrons sometimes slept in shifts and the beds never got cold.
Thousands of vagrants and day laborers lived in lodging houses amidst
vermin, filth, and disease.[14]

A reporter and a photographer from the *Sunday Call* accompanied
the tenement board inspectors in July 1904 on a house-to-house inspection. The first place visited was a four-story brick tenement house at
67 and 69 River Street. A saloon occupied the first floor front at No.
67, and a grocery store the opposite side. The buildings had neither fire
escapes nor toilets. Water closets of the "school sink" variety were provided the tenants in the enclosed court in the rear of the building. Though
this type of privy was condemned as unsanitary by the board of health,
the investigators found it very much in evidence. A sloping open sewer
drained each closet, and if the tanks had been flushed out every ten minutes
as intended, the privies would not have been as filthy as they were. The
closets, however, were connected with a water meter and consequently
were flushed only once a day. In the enclosed court, chickens were wan-
dering about, and on the roof there was a tumbledown shanty. Another
courtyard visited by the inspectors was described as "vile beyond de-
scription. Reeking with odors that almost sicken one, filled with disease germs and foul to the touch and sight . . ."[15]

The investigators then went a little down the block to a four-story
brick tenement located at 58 River Street. In the cellar of the building
there were three low, dark rooms, each occupied by a family. Naked
children and half-undressed occupants swarmed about. Underground
sleeping rooms were forbidden in the tenement house act, but in a basement at 89 River Street a table was set for a meal and a mattress was laid
out. Still, the people in the area swore that the room was only a workshop for a scissors grinder. Everywhere that the investigators found evidence of illegal occupancy there were denials from the local inhabitants.

A two-story frame shanty measuring at most ten feet by twelve feet,
which "in a respectable community would scarcely be used for a
woodshed," was found in the rear of 133 South Canal Street. In apartments at 117 South Canal Street there were "Italians and negroes ming-

ling with the greatest freedom." The courtyard separating the front and
rear buildings was wet and slimy with the excrement of chickens and
dogs. In one spot in the courtyard dirty-looking dish water was being
heated in a pail by means of a charcoal fire. The *Sunday Call* reporter
summed up the attitude of "good people" to the tenement housing problem by observing:

> Most of the dwellers in the tenement districts are foreigners, used to
> conditions at home so immeasureably worse than they find here that
> they are content to live amid such surroundings without protest.
>
> Carelessness and shiftlessness on the part of the people themselves are
> largely responsible for the . . . tenement-house sections, and things
> will not be changed until they are ordered to be changed by the
> board.[16]

In its struggles to ameliorate the housing of the poor, the Board of
Tenement House Supervision compiled a mixed record. For one thing,
the board was severely limited by lack of funds. The inspecting force
of the board during its first year comprised just nine men. At a time
before there were automobiles, this small force was expected to canvass
45,000 tenement houses in an area extending from Newark to Cape May
and to supervise in every detail the building of the approximately 1,000
new tenement houses each year.[17]

Slumlords utilized an assortment of subterfuges to evade the board's
regulations. Speculators bought run-down, violation-ridden tenements
which they "milked" and unloaded on other speculators before inspectors could catch up to them. Owners of one- and two-family houses
sought to remove their buildings from the tenement class through a
loophole in the law which defined a tenement as a building in which tenants had "a common right in the halls, stairways, yards, water-closets,
privies or some of them." A simple partition denying one or more families use of certain parts of the house would therefore free the building
of regulation. Owners of small houses who wanted to get out from under the board's control could simply limit occupancy to two families,
but then any action that reduced overcrowding was a step in the right
direction.[18]

The attitude of tenants toward housing reform furnished an object
lesson in human nature. Building inspectors were startled to find them-

selves accused of "prying" by the very persons they were trying to aid.
Despite the fact that complaints were kept confidential, fear of reprisal
silenced many tenants. Improvements ordered by the board were un-
dermined by the actions of careless tenants. Newly installed waterclosets
were allowed to become run-down and dirty, and the removal of vermin-
infested woodwork from enclosed sinks was resisted. Fire escapes, which
needed to be kept clear to permit rapid descent in an emergency, were
obstructed with brooms, mops, and other household implements. Finally, of what good were windows hidden by blinds and dark curtains?
Tenant behavior at times exasperated and incensed the board. What
the board failed to understand, however, was that much of the tenants'
conduct resulted not from an innate intractability, but rather from a need
for more storage space and a desire for privacy. The roots of the anti-
social behavior of the poor lay in their unmet needs.[19]

A losing battle was waged to upgrade old tenement houses. The owners of the buildings could not easily pass on the cost of the improvements
required by the board and, in any case, preferred to invest their money
in new housing. The requirement that every room have a window provides an example of the limitations inherent in trying to make old dwellings meet new standards of health and safety. The requirement was set
to provide railroad flats with more light and air. But the sash windows
placed in the cross partitions between the interior and exterior rooms
caught precious little fresh air and sunshine, and the inside rooms remained unpleasantly close and dark.[20] In 1909 the board admitted that
the thinness of its field force had prevented it from "reinspecting the
old buildings as frequently as might be desirable. As a consequence, the
department often finds that houses have, in some respects, reverted to
the old conditions."[21]

A class-ethnic bias is discernible in the writings of the tenement house
board supervisors. The journalists, clergymen, philanthropists, and
physicians who supported tenement house reform belonged to the middle and upper classes. The members of the board served without pay,
and all employees, except for the head, were appointed by civil service
examination. Not paying the members was supposed to keep the
board free from political influence, but it also meant that the views of
the poor were not represented. The board's clients were regarded as ig-
norant foreigners who would have to be educated for their own good
and that of the community in the American way of doing things. In-
evitably, paternalism, condescension, and class bias permeated the board's

work.[22] One can sense, for example, an undercurrent in the annual reports of the board that mendacity was to be expected of the immigrant owners of tenements and coercion might be necessary in dealing with them. On the other hand, corporations and locally prominent citizens, who made up a fair proportion of tenement house owners, simply had "not been made aware of their responsibilities,"[23] and could be expected to do the right thing when so informed.

Immigrant owners of tenement properties resisted the demands of housing inspectors for expensive renovations. The buildings in question were one- and two-family frame dwellings which immigrants had converted into tenements to supplement their incomes. The usually heavily mortgaged houses operated with tiny profit margins and little leeway for raising rents. Moreover, it hardly seemed fair to enforce the law against small operators when the reformers were willing to tolerate the basic income relationships of the society in which a wealthy minority nakedly exploited the labor of the masses. Not surprisingly, the immigrant property owner regarded the state's attempts to enforce safe living conditions as harassment, which he sought to neutralize through petty bribery and the help of the local political boss.[24]

The board had better success in supervising the building of new tenement housing. In 1911 the board was authorized to issue stop work orders on buildings with a record of serious, persistent violations. Until then the board had had its hands tied in such cases by lengthy court litigation. Fears that the stringent requirements of the tenement house act would put a crimp in new construction proved baseless. After an initial period of opposition, builders were pacified by the expanded and higher rent market which the new style apartments were able to command. Throughout the decade 1904-1914 the rate of new tenement house construction remained on a high plateau.[25]

The work of the Board of Tenement House Supervision was augmented by the activities of municipal health and building authorities. Newark housing standards were laid down in building, sanitation, plumbing, and fire codes. Though the provisions of the tenement house act were intended to be supplementary to the ordinances and duties of local governments, the real impetus to tenement house reform in Newark came from the state.[26]

In a report on housing made in 1913 by the Newark City Plan Commission, the tenement housing regulatory work of the Newark Board of

Health was criticized on several accounts. The board of health employed eighteen sanitary inspectors, "an obviously inadequate number," and displayed a "lack of aggressiveness" in initiating housing reform. Not enough original inspections were made, especially in tenement districts where immigrant tenants had not yet learned to report unsafe conditions. Record-keeping procedures were culpably negligent; for instance, no effort was made to link cases of typhoid fever with defective sanitary appliances. Fines for infractions of the law were too low to deter unscrupulous landlords, and penalties were not collected when offenders were dilatory in stopping violations. A full measure of the blame must be ascribed to the callousness of influential citizens regarding the suffering of the poor. The board, commented the City Plan Commission, needs the "aid of an enlightened public opinion which will remove political pressure and the legal handicaps which restrict the Board's effectiveness."[27] The commission concluded that under the circumstances state and local enforcement agencies were operating "as well as could be expected," and housing inspection in Newark was being performed "at least as well as in the average large American city."[28]

While the housing built under the auspices of the Board of Tenement House Supervision was a great improvement over what existed before, it is clear from the remarks of contemporary observers that the board failed to alter significantly the housing conditions of the majority of tenement dwellers.[29] One basic flaw in the tenement house law was that there was no program of publicly financed housing. The supply of decent housing thus remained dependent upon the attractiveness of new housing construction to investors and the ability of the lower class to pay for better design and new fixtures. The apartments erected under the Tenement House Act of 1904 provided sunshine, fresh air, sanitary appliances, adequate space, and fire protection, but there simply were not enough of them to go around. Moreover, with regard to one- and two-family houses, it was still possible to build and maintain dwellings which were dark, dingy, and dangerous. Finally, the moral and health concerns of reformers touched only one dimension of the housing problem. They did not speak, for example, to the need for giving support to auxiliary public services. Today, after sixty years of toil in these vineyards, the solutions to the housing problems of the poor remain as elusive as ever.[30]

The distribution of manufacturing work to be done outside the factory was a byproduct of tenement housing. Industrial homework was resorted to in the finishing or making of garments, the production of artificial flowers and cigars, and in a variety of other light industries. In some instances the contractor rented rooms in a tenement, and in other instances the work was done in private houses. The work force consisted of marginal laborers, mainly immigrant women and children who labored long hours under conditions inimical to health. Industrial homework also threatened the welfare of the community. Goods worn or consumed by the public, the principal items of manufacture, were made in an unsanitary environment, frequently by persons afflicted with acute communicable diseases. Factory owners resorted to industrial homework because it reduced their fixed costs, especially during seasonal periods of peak productivity when additional plant space was needed. An estimated 81 percent of Newark factories in 1905 engaged in the practice at one time or another. A few employers who operated entirely out of tenement sweatshops took advantage of the low overhead costs and the miserable wages paid women and children to undercut legitimate manufacturers.[31]

New Jersey's first law regulating industrial homework, enacted in 1904, required that in fourteen specified industries contractors be licensed contingent upon inspection of their employees' work premises. There were several weaknesses in the law, the most important one being that licenses were conferred for an indefinite period with no provision for reinspection.[32]

About this time the Consumer's League of New Jersey launched an imaginative attack on the industrial homework evil. Photographs prepared by the league, and displayed in tuberculosis exhibits, contrasted conditions in tenement sweatshops with those in factories whose products carried the league's label. Besides having great propaganda value, the photographs of women and children working in poor light stooped over sewing machines caused many consumers to boycott products not carrying the league's label. The league was also an adept lobbyist in the state legislature.[33]

In 1916 the New York Legislature outlawed the practice of industrial homework in several industries, causing the industries to move to nearby urban centers in New Jersey. The following year the New Jersey Legislature responded by compelling the licensing of all industrial homework contractors and by stipulating that licenses be renewed annually, also, the making of dolls and doll and infant clothing in tenements was forbidden. Though an improvement, the law was still deficient in that the exploitation of women and children in tenement sweatshops was allowed to continue.[34]

NOTES

1. Laurence Veiller, "Housing as a Factor in Health Progress in the Past Fifty Years," *A Half Century of Public Health: Jubilee Historical Volume of the American Public Health Association,* ed. Mazÿck Porcher Ravenel (New York: American Public Health Association, 1921), pp. 323-4; George Rosen, *A History of Public Health* (New York: MD Publications, Inc., 1957), p. 236; Robert H. Bremner, *From the Depths: The Discovery of Poverty in the United States* (New York: New York University Press, 1956), pp. 204-13.

2. Sam Bass Warner, Jr., *The Urban Wilderness: A History of the American City* (New York: Harper & Row, 1972), p. 201.

3. Howard D. Kramer, "History of the Public Health Movement in the United States, 1850 to 1900" (Unpublished Ph.D. diss., State University of Iowa, 1942), pp. 131-2.

4. Willard D. Price, *The Ironbound District: A Study of a District in Newark, N.J.* (Newark: The Neighborhood House, 1912), pp. 24-25. My thinking on this subject has been guided by Warner, *The Urban Wilderness,* pp. 202-5.

5. U.S. Bureau of the Census, *Eleventh Census of the United States, 1890: Report on Vital and Social Statistics,* II, 3-4; Veiller, "Housing," pp. 323-333; George B. Ford and E. P. Goodrich, *Housing Report,* [Reports of] *The City Plan Commission, Newark, N.J.* (Newark: Mathias Plum, 1913), pp. 5-6.

6. In 1900 30.2 percent of Newark families lived in one-family houses, 29.4 percent in two-family houses, 21.3 percent in three-family houses, and 19.1 percent in four- or more-family houses. 62 Cong., 1 Sess., Senate Document No. 22, *Cost of Living in American Towns,* p. 303.

7. Samuel Harry Popper, "Newark, N.J., 1870-1910: Chapters in the Evolution of an American Metropolis," (Unpublished Ph.D. diss., New York University, 1952), pp. 173-80; Ford and Goodrich, *Housing Report,* p. 1; *NJRCC,* VIII (1909), 558; N.J., Board of Tenement House Supervision, *Annual Report, 1904,* pp. 6-7 (hereinafter referred to as *ARNJBTHS*).

8. *ARNJBTHS, 1904,* p. 35.

9. *Sunday Call,* Jan. 31, 1904.

10. Popper, "Newark," p. 176. A tenement house was defined as a "house or building or portion thereof which is rented, leased, let or

hired out to be occupied or is occupied as the house or residence of three families or more living independently of each other and doing the cooking upon the premises, or by more than two families upon any floor so living and cooking, but having a common right in the halls, stairways, yards, water-closets, privies, or some of them."

11. *ARNJBTHS, 1909,* pp. 9-10; *NJRCC,* VIII (1909), 558-60.

12. The following sections are based on 62 Cong., 1 Sess., Senate Document No. 22, *Cost of Living in American Towns,* pp. 304-5; Popper, "Newark," pp. 175-80.

13. Ford and Goodrich, *Housing Report,* pp. 7-10; *NJRCC,* III (1904), 14, 19.

14. *Sunday Call,* Jan. 31, 1904.

15. Ibid., July 10, 1904.

16. Ibid.

17. *NJRCC,* VIII (1909), 558.

18. *ARNJBTHS, 1907,* p. 24, *1914,* p. 86.

19. Ibid., *1904,* p. 45, *1905,* pp. 6-7, *1911,* pp. 28-29, 31; Ford and Goodrich, *Housing Report,* pp. 17-18.

20. 62 Cong., 1 Sess., Senate Document No. 22, *Cost of Living in American Towns,* p. 305.

21. *NJRCC,* VIII (1909), 559.

22. Warner, *Urban Wilderness,* p. 220; Miles W. Beemer, "The City and Housing," Proceedings of the Fifth National Conference on Housing (Providence, 1916), *Housing Problems in America,* pp. 352-7.

23. *ARNJBTHS,* 1906, pp. 22, 24-25.

24. Warner, *Urban Wilderness,* p. 220.

25. *ARNJBTHS, 1911,* pp. 5, 12.

26. Ford and Goodrich, *Housing Report,* pp. 26-27.

27. Ibid., pp. 27-28, 41-42, 47-49.

28. Ibid., p. 49.

29. See, for instance, *NJRCC,* VIII (1909), 510-3.

30. Warner, *Urban Wilderness,* p. 224; Ford and Goodrich, Housing Report, p. 25.

31. Philip Charles Newman, *The Labor Legislation of New Jersey* (Washington: American Council on Public Affairs, 1943), p. 109; Annie S. Daniels, "The Causes, Evils, and Remedy for Tenement-Housing Manufacturing," 15th International Congress on Hygiene and Demography, *Transactions,* Vol. III (Washington, 1912), 1011-4.

32. Susanna P. Zwemmer, "History of Consumer's League of New Jersey (1900-1950)," pp. 12-13, Rutgers University, Consumer's League of New Jersey MSS, Box 5; National Consumer's League, *Annual Report*

for the Year Ending March 1, 1906, p. 16; Elizabeth B. Butler, "Factory Work in Newark Homes," National Consumer's League, *Annual Report for the Year Ending March 1, 1906,* pp. 29-34.

33. Zwemmer, "History of Consumer's League," pp. 12-13.

34. Newman, *Labor Legislation,* pp. 109-10.

Conclusion

A pervasive business ethic permeated the marrow of the Newark community. Newark's proudest boast was the ingenuity and manufacturing skills of its citizens. As a mark of the esteem which Newark accorded its mechanics, in 1890 a bronze statue was unveiled in Washington Park of Seth Boyden, an artisan whose inventions were instrumental in the city's early growth. The statue portrayed him in his work clothes standing next to an anvil. On national holidays and on municipal anniversaries speakers elaborated on the theme that Newark was a community of manufacturers, a workshop for the nation. In 1872 the Newark Industrial Exposition was opened to advertise the city's wares. The event marked the first time an American city had sponsored an exhibit limited to its own products. The exposition was open from August 20 to October 11 and attracted upward of 130,000 persons. Encouraged by the large, enthusiastic crowds who attended the fair, the exposition's sponsors staged encores in the three succeeding years.[1]

During the last decades of the nineteenth century a rash of souvenirs, pamphlets, and books was published extolling the advantages of Newark. Columns of statistics furnishing the capital investment and the number of persons employed in Newark enterprises suggested a crude equating of industrial growth with community welfare. Histories of Newark and Essex County recounted in detail the industrial development of Newark. Both scholarly local histories and frank municipal advertisements contained glossy photographs of the city's benefactors. The finely-tailored cloth and stern countenances seen in these photographs convey an image of men certain of their station in life and at one with the world. The business mentality was shared by clergymen and newspaper editors and was even concurred in to a startling degree by trade unionists. The persons who counted in Newark agreed that continued business prosperity assured the making of the best of all possible worlds.

On public health questions that directly impinged upon the city's economic prosperity, the Newark Board of Trade gave unstinting support. Thus the board played a leading role in improving drainage, in obtaining pure water, in reclaiming the meadows, and in cleansing the Passaic River. It was a different story when the returns from public health were less obvious or when their cost would have to be borne by businessmen. Thus the board did not participate in the movement for the reduction of infant and maternal mortality and was less than enthusiastic about the Tenement House Act of 1904 (though eager to share in the credit for its passage).[2] Moreover, the board opposed industrial hygiene reform. In 1913 it appealed to the legislature to delete "certain burdensome provisions" from the Sanitary and Engineering Industrial Standards issued by the commissioner of labor which, it protested, were "being forced in a drastic way by [Department of Labor] inspectors."[3] The board also indicated its desire of seeing the department reorganized.[4]

Though responsive to the need for modernization of municipal services, Newark community leaders could not conceive that an inordinate share of the burdens of industrialization fell on the shoulders of the working class. Labor strife and other social problems confronting the community had no place in the litany of civic boosters. Critics who questioned the traditional wisdom were rebuffed. The intolerance shown dissenters is revealed in the reaction of businessmen and clergymen to a survey undertaken in 1912 by Willard D. Price, a social worker in the Neighborhood [Settlement] House of the "Ironbound" district.

Price cut through the pretense that shrouded Newark's worst slum. The tone of the report was established in the opening paragraph in which "Ironbound" was described as

> a district of industrial uproar, drifting smoke, heavy atmosphere, dangerous acid fumes and unforgettable odors. Its people are a hodgepodge of nationalities, speaking many old-world tongues, and making pathetic efforts to adjust to their new and unwholesome American surroundings.[5]

The district's dearth of "positive" recreational outlets led to patronage of less reputable facilities. About the only place where workers could relax amidst the good cheer of friends was the neighborhood saloon. There were 122 saloons to choose from, one for every seven residential buildings. In the dance halls couples were observed in close sensual embrace doing the "Grizzly Bear." While he found "little distinctly immoral dancing," Price was struck by the absence of any "good dancing." Three gambling houses operated in open defiance of the law.[6]

Dilapidated one-family frame houses that had been converted into tenements comprised the neighborhood's basic housing unit. "The inevitable results," reported Price, "are constant discomfort, the spread of tuberculosis, the breaking down of family life, lack of privacy, and widespread immorality."[7] In tenements of less than four stories, combustible wooden staircases were used as fire escapes. Several old houses did not have water and sewer connections, which Price attributed to the discretionary powers granted the Newark Board of Health in enforcing the Sanitary Code.

> The opportunities afforded by such powers for political and commercial favoritism are obvious, and it is also obvious to anyone living in "The Ironbound District" that such opportunities are not always lost.[8]

Price censured the city for having closed its eyes to the industrial abuses that abounded in Newark. He found the "Ironbound" community "seething with resentment of industrial cruelty and oppression."[9] One firm was notorious for its frequency of accidents.

> So many times a week is the ambulance called to the door of this plant that it is a common saying when the ambulance bell is heard clanging down the street, 'One more on ————'s junk heap.'[10]

Stating that the need was urgent, Price recommended that an inquiry be undertaken into the wage structure and working conditions of "Ironbound" factories.[11]

The survey came under attack from the Manufacturers and Merchants Association of New Jersey. J. A. Roney, the Association's secretary, answered Price in a pamphlet wherein he cautioned that every large city had its poor district "to which present day social workers affix the term 'The Slums.' " He invoked the Scriptures in defense of the status quo by reminding his readers "that the greatest Social Worker of all said: 'The poor ye have always with you.' " Unaware of the irony of his words, Roney found contentment among "those whose lives must be eked out

near to where they are employed, amidst the drum and grind of industries, smoking chimneys, [and] the dust-laden atmosphere."[12]

Roney attributed the squalor of the area to the sloth and improvi-
dence of the newer immigrant groups and admonished them that "a man's
home is just what he wills it to be." He wrote admiringly of the industry
and thrift of the earlier Irish and German stock, and stated that it would
probably take the present residents of "Ironbound" several years to shed
their native ways.[13]

Roney's comments were liberally laced with disparaging remarks about
college-educated social uplifters. He accused Price of setting class against
class and of planning "to revolutionize everything." He implied that
Price was wet behind the ears, showed no understanding of human nature,
and was afflicted with a savior complex.[14] Included in Roney's reply was
a blunt warning that the survey would not find favor among "the large
manufacturing concerns of this part of the city upon which social workers find themselves financially dependent."[15] (The headquarters of the
Manufacturers and Merchants Association of New Jersey was on downtown Broad Street on the periphery of the "Ironbound" district.)

Four letters highly critical of Price from clergymen in the district were
included in an appendix to Roney's comments.[16] The clergymen defended the social facilities provided by Ironbound churches for their
parishioners and stated that if persons went instead to saloons and dance
halls it reflected on their upbringing. Price was denounced for under-
mining obedience to home and church and for making residents "feel
that the only thing needed for their uplifting is dancing, amusements
and free social intercourse."[17] The allegations made by Price, however,
were left unanswered.

Urban public health reform has thus far largely escaped the purview
of historians of the Progressive Period.[18] Yet the Progressives knew that
the humane and just society they envisioned would remain a shibboleth
so long as men were stalked by illness. The environmental conditions
that sapped vitality and destroyed health were never far from the con-
sciousness of reformers who worked among the poor. Seizing upon the
revolutionary discoveries made in sanitary engineering and medical
science, the Progressives effected a profound reduction in morbidity
and mortality.

Conversely, Progressivism left a deep imprint upon the public health
movement. Progressivism was linked to public health reform in both obvious and subtle ways. Campaigns to rid the body politic of boss rule

and other impurities found their counterparts in the cleansing of the environment of filth and dirt. On the state level, Progressives fought to protect workers against industrial hazards and to improve tenement housing. The need to protect the health of mothers and children was just one of many fruitful ideas to spring from Progressive reexamination of traditional attitudes toward child behavior and the role of women in society (others included: progressive education, child labor legislation, new methods of treating juvenile offenders, and the granting of the franchise to women). Finally, the Progressive spirit manifested itself in increased government expenditures for public health and in the desire for expertise in the administration of public services.

Unlike the great social insurance measures that were paternalistically bestowed upon the German people in the late nineteenth century, Progressivism was a grass-roots phenomenon. The mainsprings of reform in the United States were local and voluntary. The initiative was taken simultaneously across the nation by private citizens in revolt against the excesses of the "Gilded Age."

If industrialization had thrown the existing order out of kilter, it had also created an economic surplus which could be channeled into righting social wrongs. Philanthropic groups and voluntary health associations multiplied. Freed from the around-the-clock drudgery of household chores, middle and upper-class women became active in public affairs. In organizations such as The Neighborhood House, the Essex County Welfare Committee, the Essex County Medical Milk Commission, the Newark Anti-Tuberculosis Association, the National Consumer's League, and the Visiting Nurse Association, civic-minded citizens supported and extended public health reform. At times these groups acted in an ancillary capacity to local health authorities, while at other times they were gadflies. Free of the political constraints that bound public officials, voluntary public health associations were uniquely suited to spotlight neglected problems and to pioneer in public health.

Within Newark governmental circles, Progressivism manifested itself principally in the desire for efficiency. The suffering of the urban masses brought on by unbridled industrialization (usually referred to as the "social question" by Progressives) played second fiddle to the maintenance of a healthy business climate that would attract new industry to Newark. Reformers were tolerated so long as they did not challenge the basic tenets of laissez-faire capitalism. The Newark Board of Health, which was recruited from the business community and its professional allies, fully accepted these institutional arrangements. Thus the board emphasized professionalism in the operation of the health department but was unwilling to challenge the vested interests of Newark businessmen in unsafe factories and run-down tenements. Only in its milk and infant welfare work did the board evince a deep, humanitarian concern for the poor.

Many diverse individuals contributed to public health reform in Newark. A physician in private practice, Henry L. Coit, played a prominent role in improving the wholesomeness and safety of the milk supply, not only for Newark, but for all American communities. Charles V. Craster, Julius Levy, and other zealous officials kept Newark abreast of new trends in public health. An exposé by the *Newark Evening News* focused attention on the city's poor milk supply and led to the creation of a milk division within the health department.

The Essex County Medical Society, which earlier had largely ignored the county's urban health needs, began to involve itself in public health issues. Under the aegis of the American Medical Association, the medical profession was becoming a powerful force in American life. The spectacular achievements of medicine in the late nineteenth and early twentieth centuries enhanced the prestige of the profession and enabled it to act more boldly than it had in the past.[19] The Essex County Medical Society responded to the challenge by lending its support to local health authorities. Within a few years standing committees were established in the society on milk, tuberculosis, public health, public health education, and sexual hygiene. The society was especially active in arranging public lectures on sex. By calling attention to the widespread existence of venereal disease at a time when sex was a taboo subject, the society performed a great public service.[20]

By 1919 most major acute infectious diseases, with the exception of respiratory diseases, had been brought under control. Intestinal infections (typhoid fever, cholera), diseases spread by insects (malaria, yellow fever, typhus, bubonic plague), and maladies for which vaccines or antitoxins had been found (smallpox, rabies, diphtheria) had largely become a thing of the past. Substantial progress had also been made in areas of public health where education and socioeconomic conditions are paramount, as in tuberculosis and infant mortality. Newark's death rate in 1922 was a mere 12.1 per 1,000 population, 60 percent less than it was in 1890.

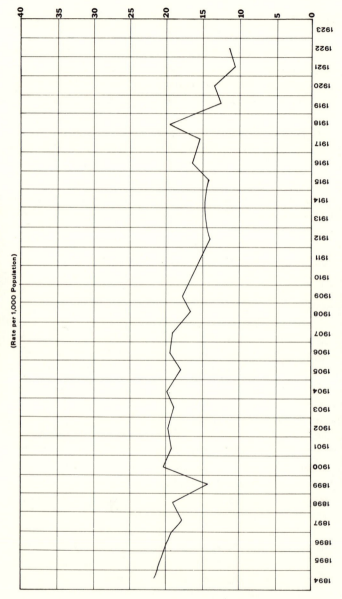

PLATE VI

NEWARK'S ANNUAL DEATH RATE, 1894—1923

(Rate per 1,000 Population)

SOURCE: NEWARKS OWN HEALTH RECORD (NEWARK: MUTUAL Benefit Life Insurance Co.,1923),p.5

NOTES

1. John T. Cunningham, *Newark* (Newark: The New Jersey Historical Society, 1966), pp. 170-6.

2. Contrast *NJRCC,* III (1904), 180-1 with *Annual Report of the Board of Trade, 1905,* p. 31.

3. *Annual Report of the Board of Trade, 1913,* p. 43.

4. Ibid., *1914,* p. 160.

5. Willard D. Price, *The Ironbound District: A Study of a District in Newark, N.J.* (Newark: The Neighborhood House, 1912), p. 3.

6. Ibid., pp. 4-12.

7. Ibid., p. 23.

8. Ibid., pp. 24-25.

9. Ibid., p. 25.

10. Ibid., p. 26.

11. Ibid., p. 25.

12. Joseph A. Roney, *Uplifting Down-Neck* (n.p., 1912), p. 1.

13. Ibid., pp. 3-13.

14. Ibid., pp. 14-15.

15. Ibid., p. 1.

16. Ibid., pp. 23-30.

17. Ibid.

18. However, there are books on tenement housing, social work, the settlement movement, and national health legislation during the Progressive Era that touch on urban health campaigns.

19. James Gordon Burrow, *A.M.A.: Voice of American Medicine,* (Baltimore: Johns Hopkins Press, 1963), p. 28.

20. *Minutes ECMS,* IV (1904), 3, V (1911), 25-26, (1912), 24-26, V (1913), 12-14, 24-26; Thomas N. Gray, "The Social Evil and its Relationship to Public Health," *NJRCC,* IX (June-July 1911), 5-14.

Appendix

APPENDIX

MORTALITY IN NEWARK FROM ACUTE COMMUNICABLE DISEASES ALONG WITH OTHER SELECTED VITAL STATISTICS,

SECTION A: 1879 — 1880 — 1889

	1879-80	80-81	81-82	82-83	83-84	84-85	85-86	86-87	87-88	88-89
POPULATION	—	136508	—	—	—	—	—	—	152988	—
DEATHS	3116	2553	2884	3912	3480	3372	—	3663	3734	4133
DEATH RATE (per 1000 pop)	—	—	—	—	25.49	24.70	24.33	23.90	24.40	27.02
BIRTHS	3567	3518	3737	3646	3952	3889	3494	4311	4540	4751
INFANT MORTALITY	757	641	654	871	830	836	885	897	948	1107
INFANT MORTALITY RATE (per 1000 bir.) [a]	207.00	182.21	175.01	238.89	210.02	214.97	253.29	208.07	208.81	233.00
CHOLERA	0	0	0	0	0	0	0	0	0	0
DIPHTHERIA AND CROUP	214	144	231	309	182	176	438	257	226	397
ERYSIPELAS	18	5	20	10	14	6	8	20	13	20
INFANTILE PARALYSIS										
MALARIA	60	48	65	42	30	28	31	33	17	41
MEASLES	28	3	2	60	8	48	16	14		10
MENINGITIS										
CEREBROSPINAL MENINGITIS										
RESPIRATORY DISEASES	309	308	346	490	404	407	410	415	380	483
BRONCHITIS										
INFLUENZA										
PNEUMONIA										
OTHER RESPIRATORY DISEASES										
SCARLET FEVER	120	35	42	310	271	79	68	22	21	34
SMALLPOX	0	0	4	19	1	0	0	1	2	0
TUBERCULOSIS	448	396	453	551	542	486	565	546	649	557
TYPHOID FEVER	65	72	51	97	89	87	94	85	84	76
TYPHUS	0	0	0	0	0	0	0	0	0	0
WHOOPING COUGH	44	11	4	47	37	6	21	44	21	19

[a] Computations by the author.

SOURCE: Annual Reports of the New Jersey Board of Health. Statistics are for the period July 1 — June 30.

	1889-90	90-91	91-92	92-93	93-94	94-95	95-96	96-97	97-98
POPULATION	166172	181518	186598	193366	198636	204902	—	222601	229396
DEATHS	4258	4948	4420	5641	4900	4760	4643	4628	4496
DEATH RATE (per 1000 pop)	23.59	27.25	23.69	29.17	24.60	22.68	—	20.79	19.60
BIRTHS	4920	4902	4810	4927	5410	5336	4684	4364	4754
INFANT MORTALITY	1157	1327	1156	1520	1350	1253	1129	1105	1153
INFANT MORTALITY RATE (per 1000 bir.) [a]	235.16	270.71	240.33	308.30	249.54	234.82	241.38	253.22	242.55
CHOLERA									
DIPHTHERIA AND CROUP	343	314	196	219	275	173	256	330	177
ERYSIPELAS	14	12	12	18	17	15	17	21	15
INFANTILE PARALYSIS									
MALARIA	22	36	32	39	17	15	13	13	17
MEASLES	16	64	15	88	7	48	12	97	35
MENINGITIS									
CEREBROSPINAL MENINGITIS									
RESPIRATORY DISEASES	465	693	597	876	731	696	740	663	630
BRONCHITIS									
INFLUENZA									
PNEUMONIA									
OTHER RESPIRATORY DISEASES									
SCARLET FEVER	48	67	45	302	153	122	33	22	45
SMALLPOX				14	5	2	19		
TUBERCULOSIS	617	661	634	624	617	608	595	584	581
TYPHOID FEVER	131	194	134	153	63	43	43	61	44
TYPHUS									
WHOOPING COUGH	50	47	52	20	31	28	46	33	59

[a] Computations by the author

SOURCE: Annual Reports of the New Jersey Board of Health. Statistics are for the period July 1 —June 30.

SECTION C: 1898 – 1908

	1898	1899	1900	1901	1902	1903	1904	1905	1906	1907	1908
POPULATION	235000	240000	246070	250000	255000	266000	272000	283289	290000	300000	305000
DEATHS	4303	3537	5000	4806	4943	4923	5378	5025	5551	5724	5207
DEATH RATE (per 1000pop)	18.30	18.90	20.34	19.22	19.38	18.50	19.77	17.74	19.14	19.08	17.07
BIRTHS	5188	6721	6117	6016	6439	7041	7036	7110	7649	8379	8912
INFANT MORTALITY	—	989	1122	1086	1109	969	1121	1026	1196	1133	1169
INFANT MORTALITY RATE (per 1000 bir.) [a]	—	133.61	185.04	180.67	172.17	137.61	159.32	144.30	157.80	135.22	131.17
CHOLERA	0	0	0	0	0	0	0	0	0	0	0
DIPHTHERIA AND CROUP	133	124	139	103	105	120	150	110	99	95	66
ERYSIPELAS	—	—	—	—	8	20	25	21	16	32	26
INFANTILE PARALYSIS											
MALARIA	—	16	—	10	13	5	9	5	7	9	0
MEASLES	—	6	56	13	51	2	39	13	37	18	22
MENINGITIS	—	201	63	159	—	—	129	—	131	167	87
CEREBROSPINAL MENINGITIS	—	—	—	—	156	147	51	90	20	38	11
RESPIRATORY DISEASES											
BRONCHITIS	—	118	120	157	108	108	146	113	97	123	80
INFLUENZA	—	—	64	25	13	—	25	19	15	35	26
PNEUMONIA	—	477	616	421	522	524	654	485	675	584	556
OTHER RESPIRATORY DISEASES	—	—	58	74	51	32	44	38	32	44	38
SCARLET FEVER	15	34	55	23	46	71	120	45	34	41	89
SMALLPOX	0	0	1	71	187	3	0	0	0	0	0
TUBERCULOSIS	611	624	680	640	660	718	775	781	851	850	795
TYPHOID FEVER	41	66	50	57	47	3	40	40	50	69	35
TYPHUS	0	0	0	0	0	0	0	0	0	0	0
WHOOPING COUGH	—	21	41	29	41	44	13	45	82	28	24

[a] Computations by the author.

SOURCE: Annual reports of the Newark Board of Health

SECTION D: 1909 – 1918

	1909	1910	1911	1912	1913	1914	1915	1916	1917	1918
POPULATION	311000	347469	352000	370000	380000	395000	375000	385000	405000	430000
DEATHS	5529	5784	5337	5423	5562	5809	5218	6357	6205	8483
DEATH RATE (per 1000pop)	17.77	16.64	15.16	14.65	14.63	14.70	14.35	16.50	15.30	19.72
BIRTHS	9583	10289	10898	10845	10810	11478	10955	11466	11824	11601
INFANT MORTALITY	1111	1242	1069	1076	999	1122	935	1026	1038	1215
INFANT MORTALITY RATE (per 1000 bir.) [a]	116.98	120.71	98.09	99.71	92.41	97.75	85.35	89.46	87.87	104.65
CHOLERA	–	–	–	–	–	–	–	–	–	–
DIPHTHERIA AND CROUP	105	104	74	91	110	41	44	57	50	82
ERYSIPELAS	11	27	21	31	39	33	16	16	–	–
INFANTILE PARALYSIS			3		2	1	10	376	11	6
MALARIA	1	4	3	2	1	0	1	1	0	0
MEASLES	33	32	8	27	12	44	19	102	5	20
MENINGITIS	92	91	73	58	47	54	43	75	113	80
CEREBROSPINAL MENINGITIS	7	1	5	5	8	8	14	22	68	45
RESPIRATORY DISEASES	–	–	–	–	–	–	–	–	–	–
BRONCHITIS	80	98	78	75	81	80	50	137	155	178
INFLUENZA	22	31	28	18	12	16	–	45	24	1387
PNEUMONIA	670	705	623	657	579	788	567	761	764	498
OTHER RESPIRATORY DISEASES	44	52	40	40	45	50	66	180	137	92
SCARLET FEVER	70	39	21	11	26	51	6	7	3	11
SMALLPOX	1	–	–	–	–	–	–	–	–	–
TUBERCULOSIS	764	812	707	597	733	776	835	783	820	798
TYPHOID FEVER	39	44	37	26	30	26	11	23	17	15
TYPHUS	–	–	–	–	–	–	–	–	–	–
WHOOPING COUGH	27	45	21	9	27	19	26	25	60	51

[a] Computations by the author.

SOURCE: Annual reports of the Newark Board of Health

171

A Note on the Sources

I. SECONDARY SOURCES

More has probably been written about the history of medicine than the history of any other profession. The development of public health from the earliest civilizations to the present is described in George Rosen, *A History of Public Health* (New York: MD Publications, Inc., 1957); Harry Wain, *A History of Preventive Medicine* (Springfield, Illinois: Charles C. Thomas, 1970); and Charles Wilcocks, *Medical Advance, Public Health and Social Evolution* (Oxford: Pergamon Press, 1965). The writings of Richard H. Shryock explain the evolution of modern medicine and relate significant aspects of American medical developments. Books written by Shryock include: *The Development of Modern Medicine: An Interpretation of the Social and Scientific Factors Involved* (rev. ed.; New York: Alfred A. Knopf, 1957); *Medicine in America: Historical Essays* (Baltimore: The Johns Hopkins Press, 1966); and *The National Tuberculosis Association, 1904-1954: A Study of the Voluntary Health Movement in the United States* (New York: National Tuberculosis Association, 1957). Wilson G. Smillie, *Public Health, Its Promise for the Future: A Chronicle of the Development of Public Health in the United States, 1607-1914* (New York: The Macmillan Co., 1955), though limited in perspective, is rich in detail. Kenneth F. Maxcy and Milton J. Rosenau, *Preventive Medicine and Public Health,* ed. Philip E. Sartwell (9th ed., rev. and enl.; New York: Appleton-Century-Crofts, 1965), provides scientific knowledge of communicable diseases and can be easily understood by the layman. The first edition of this classic textbook, written by Rosenau and published in 1913, gives the most advanced view of public health for its time. Accounts of the growth of public health work in the United States written by participants in the movement are found in the fifty-year histories (1871-1921) contained in Mazÿck Porcher Ravenel (ed.), *A Half Century of Public Health: Jubilee Historical Volume of the American Public Health Association* (New York: American Public Health Association, 1921).

There are, however, few histories of public health in American cities, and most of these are limited to the colonial and pre-Civil War periods. Included in this category are two fine studies: John Duffy, *A History of Public Health in New York City, 1625-1866* (New York: Russell Sage Foundation, 1968); and John B. Blake, *Public Health in the Town of Boston: 1630-1822* (Cambridge: Harvard University Press, 1959). James H. Cassedy, *Charles V. Chapin and the Public Health Movement* (Cambridge: Harvard University Press, 1962), narrates the life of one of the nation's leading public health figures around the turn of the twentieth century, who for many years served as health officer of Providence. Thomas N. Bonner, *Medicine in Chicago, 1850-1950: A Chapter in the Social and Scientific Development of a City* (Madison, Wisconsin: The American Historical Research Center, Inc., 1957) is principally concerned with the response of organized medicine to the problems confronting an indigent and aging population. William T. Howard, Jr., *Public Health Administration and the Natural History of Disease in Baltimore, Maryland: 1797-1920* (Washington: Carnegie Institution of Washington, 1924) is detailed but dated and unanalytical. A number of state public health studies touch upon urban public health problems of this period, notably Philip D. Jordan, *The People's Health: A History of Public Health in Minnesota to 1948* (Saint Paul, Minn.: Minnesota Historical Society, 1953); and Barbara G. Rosenkrantz, *Public Health and the State: Changing Views in Massachusetts, 1842-1936* (Cambridge: Harvard University Press, 1972).

Several books have been written on the history of medicine in New Jersey. An excellent overview of the subject is provided in David L. Cowen, *Medicine and Health in New Jersey: A History*, Vol. XVI of *The New Jersey Historical Society Series*, eds. Richard M. Huber and Wheaton J. Lane (Princeton, N. J.: D. Van Nostrand Co., Inc., 1964). Also useful are Fred B. Rogers, *Help Bringers: Versatile Physicians of New Jersey* (New York: Vantage Press, Inc., 1961); and Fred B. Rogers and A. Reasoner Sayre, *The Healing Art: A History of the Medical Society of New Jersey* (Trenton, N. J.: The Medical Society of New Jersey, 1966).

Historians and social scientists did not pay much attention to Newark until the racial explosion of the 1960s made the city's name synonymous with urban sickness. Consequently, many important aspects of the city's development are only now being explored. For background on Newark I relied heavily on two works: John T. Cunningham, *Newark* (Newark: The New Jersey Historical Society, 1966), a popularly written and optimistic account of the city's growth from 1666-1966; and Samuel H. Popper, "Newark, N.J., 1870-1910: Chapters in the Evolution of an American Metropolis," (Unpublished Ph.D. Diss., New York University, 1952), which focuses on business developments and municipal services. Other than that, the materials for the study are drawn from primary sources. In the late nineteenth and early twentieth centuries several locally sponsored histories and guidebooks proclaiming the greatness of Newark were published. The books feature histories of Newark business firms along with biographical sketches of their founders. Self-congratulatory in tone, they ignore the darker side of Newark's history.

II. MEDICAL REFERENCE WORKS

Medical history has its own specialized reference works which the researcher would do well to familiarize himself with before beginning his labors. Happily the task is made easier by an excellent guide: National Library Association, *Medical Reference Works, 1679-1966, A Selected Bibliography,* eds. John B. Blake and Charles Roos (Chicago: Medical Library Association, 1967). Another research aid which every medical historian should know is United States Army-Surgeon General's Office, *Index Catalogue of the Library,* 1880-1961, 58 vols. in 4 series. While the *Index Catalogue* has many uses, its main value for me was in locating pertinent journal articles published outside New Jersey. There are three good current bibliographies in the history of medicine: *Current Work in the History of Medicine,* a quarterly published by the Wellcome Historical Medical Library; a "Bibliography of the History of Medicine in the United States and Canada" has been published annually by the *Bulletin of the History of Medicine* since 1940; and an annual *Bibliography of the History of Medicine,* published by the National Library of Medicine (Vol. I, 1965-).

III. PRINTED SOURCE MATERIALS

For a city of its size, Newark's New Jersey Reference Division of its Public Library houses one of the best local history collections in the nation. Though the division's materials are well catalogued, a search of the stacks uncovered many materials that in all probability would not have been found otherwise. Among the items found were local histories, handbooks, guides, reminiscences of Newark, and pamphlets of various kinds. Some materials, especially reprints of articles written by Drs. Henry L. Coit and Julius Levy, were located in other historical and medical repositories in the Newark-New York area and in the National Library of Medicine in Bethesda.

A. Newspapers

As government documents often shy away from controversy, newspapers are indispensable for uncovering the story behind the event. For example, the annual reports of the Newark Board of Health do not mention the board's reorganization in 1915, much less the board's malfeasance, which lay behind it. Much of the information for this study was obtained by going through the complete issues of the *Newark Evening News* and the *Sunday Call* for the years 1895-1918.

B. Reports, Transactions, and Proceedings

In both England and the United States voluntary health organizations have played a key role in promoting public health reform. Business and professional groups have sometimes supported and sometimes opposed the initiatives of public health leaders. The activities of these organizations, as discovered in their annual statements, shed considerable light on public health developments in Newark. Used in this study were: American Association of Medical Milk Commissions, *Proceedings of the Annual Conference,* 1907, 1910; Babies Hospital of the City of Newark, N. J., *Annual Report,* 1897, 1898-1899, 1900, 1903, 1908-1909, 1911; (Newark) Board of Trade, *Annual Report* (Yearbook), 1895, 1897, 1899-1900, 1902-1911, 1913-1916; Bureau of Associated Charities of Newark, New Jersey, *Annual Report,* 1897-1910; Essex County Medical Milk Commission, *Annual Report,* 1893-1916; Medical Society of New Jersey, *Transactions,* 1807-1974; New Jersey Association for the Prevention and

Relief of Tuberculosis, *Annual Report,* 1906-1907, 1907-1908, 1908-1909, 1911-1912, 1912-1913; New Jersey Mosquito Extermination Association, *Proceedings of the Annual Meeting,* 1914-1918; Newark Anti-Tuberculosis Association (Committee of One Hundred), *Annual Report,* 1909-1910, 1911-1912, 1912-1913.

C. Periodicals and Articles

Numerous articles were found in *Transactions of the Medical Society of New Jersey* and New Jersey Board of Health, *Annual Report,* two treasure stores of information for historians of various persuasions still virtually untapped. Besides accounts of sickness, the journals contain information on social and economic conditions and furnish demographic data. Also used were: Miles W. Beemer, "The City and Housing," Proceedings of the Fifth National Conference on Housing (Providence, 1916), *Housing Problems in America,* pp. 352-7; *Clean Milk: A Bi-Monthly Bulletin Issued by the Medical Milk Commission of Essex County, N. J.,* 1916-1926; Henry L. Coit, "A Plan to Procure Cows' Milk Designed for Clinical Purposes: Paper Read before the Practitioner's Club, Newark, N. J., January, 1893," *Report of the* [N. J.] *Dairy Commissioner for the Year 1893,* pp. 10-18; "A Crusader and His Accomplishments, the Story of a Life Dedicated to Milk Improvement," *Certified Milk: Official Publication of American Association of Medical Milk Commissions, Inc., and Certified Milk Producers of America, Inc.,* XXIV, No. 8 (1949), 2-3, 14; Annie S. Daniels, "The Causes, Evils, and Remedy for Tenement-House Manufacturing," 15th International Congress on Hygiene and Demography, *Transactions,* Vol. III (Washington, 1912), 1,011-1,014; Earnest D. Eaton, "Forty Years of Progress in the Control of Tuberculosis," [N.J.] *Public Health News,* XXVII (Dec. 1946), 179-81; James Ford, "Housing Conditions as Factors in the Production of Disease," Proceedings of the Fifth National Conference on Housing (Providence, 1916), *Housing Problems in America,* pp. 190-7; "From Certification to Pasteurization," *American Journal of Public Health,* XLIV (1954), 929-30; Rosary S. Gilheany, "Early Newark Hospitals," *Proceedings of the New Jersey Historical Society,* LXI (Jan. 1965), 10-24; Elisha Harris, "Report on the Public Health Service in the Principal Cities, and the Progress of the Sanitary Works in the United States," American Public Health Association, *Public Health Reports and Papers,* II (1874-1875), 151-82; "Henry Leber Coit Memorial," *The Hospital Herald: Periodical*

of the Babies Hospital, Newark, N.J., XX, No. 2 (April 1917); H. C. H.
Herold, "Newark's Diphtheria Antitoxin Plant—Its Results and Costs,"
Annual Report of the Newark Board of Health, 1900, pp. 29-33; H. C.
H. Herold, " Report on Typhoid Fever, Newark, N. J.: 1898-1899,"
American Public Health Association, *Public Health Reports and Papers,*
XXV (1899), 172-6; Daniel Jacobson, "The Pollution Problem of the
Passaic River," *Proceedings of the New Jersey Historical Society,* LIV
(July 1958), pp. 186-98; Howard D. Kramer, "The Beginnings of the
Public Health Movement in the United States," *Bulletin of the History
of Medicine,* XXI (May-June 1947), 352-76; Howard D. Kramer, "The
Germ Theory and the Early Public Health Program in the United States,"
Bulletin of the History of Medicine, XXII (May-June 1948), 233-47;
"Meadowlands Issue, Parts 1 and 2," *Newark Commerce: Newark As-
sociation of Commerce and Industry, Newark, N. J.,* VII, No. 5 (Nov.
1962), VIII, No. 1 (Spring 1963); Mildred V. Naylor, "Henry Leber
Coit: A Biographical Sketch," *Bulletin of the History of Medicine,* XII,
No. 2 (1942), 367-76; *New Jersey Review of Charities and Corrections,
1902-1912; Newark Athletic Club News,* Feb. 1921; "Passaic Valley
Trunk Sewer Completed," *The American City Magazine* (Oct. 1924),
pp. 315-18; Joseph A. Vasselli, "A Pestilence Census-Taker in New
Jersey," *Bulletin of the History of Medicine,* XXV (1951), 354-8; J.
Ralph Van Duyne, "Eight Years Operation of Passaic Valley Sewer,"
Engineering News-Record (Oct. 13, 1932), pp. 440-2; and Manfred J.
Wasserman, "Henry L. Coit and the Certified Milk Movement in the
Development of Modern Pediatrics," *Bulletin of the History of Med-
icine,* XLVI, No. 4 (July-Aug. 1972), 359-90.

D. Government Publications

Government documents provided the lion's share of the materials
for the study. While the *Annual Report* of the Newark Board of Health
was the major source, relevant materials were also found in the records
of other municipal departments. The annual reports of city agencies
were usually published in a single bound volume under the title: Newark,
*The Mayor's Message, Together with the Reports of the City Officers of
the City of Newark, N. J.,* [date] . A few nonserial publications were
used as well. Because cities are creatures of state governments, state
documents were used extensively. The state's role in determining the
course of public health in Newark was especially important in tenement

housing, industrial hygiene, and matters of environmental sanitation requiring regional solutions, A valuable guide to New Jersey State records
is provided in Adelaide R. Hasse, *Index of Economic Materials in Documents of New Jersey, 1799-1904* (Baltimore: Carnegie Institution of
Washington, Lord Baltimore Press, 1908), a rather unfortunate title that
masks the broad scope of this work. A small number of Essex County
records were consulted on the work of the Soho Isolation Hospital and
the activities of the county mosquito extermination commission. The
United States census reports for 1880, 1890, and 1900 contain mortality statistics of American cities along with comments and descriptive
materials. Recognizing the need for up-to-date statistics, the census
bureau in 1901 began to publish annual *Mortality Statistics.* Other federal records used include: U. S. Senate, 62 Cong., 1st Sess., Senate Document No. 22, pt. 4, *Cost of Living in American Towns, Report of
an Inquiry by the Board of Trade of London into Working Class Rents,
Housing, and Retail Prices Together with Rates of Wages in Certain Occupations in the Principal Industrial Towns of the United States of
America* (Washington: Government Printing Office, 1911); U. S. Supreme
Court, October Term, 1916, *The People of the State of New York, Com-
plainants, v. State of New Jersey and Passaic Valley Sewerage Commissioners, Defendents,* 5 vols.

IV. DISSERTATIONS

Samuel H. Popper's dissertation, as already noted, describes Newark's
development in the years 1870-1910. Howard D. Kramer, "History of
the Public Health Movement in the United States, 1850-1900" (Unpublished Ph.D. diss., State University of Iowa, 1942), is a well-written account of public health theory and practice ending with the advent of
the germ theory of disease. Dorothy T. Scanlon, "The Public Health
Movement in Boston, 1870-1910" (Unpublished Ph.D. diss., Boston,
University, 1956), introduces the subject but needs to be more fully
developed.

V. MANUSCRIPTS

I did not find any manuscript records of the Newark Board of Health.
This, however, may not be as damaging to the work's value as first

feared. After comparing the manuscript minutes of the Massachusetts Department of Public Health meetings with its published *Reports,* Professor Barbara G. Rosenkrantz concluded that the manuscripts added little to the official record. Also, the meetings of the Newark Board of Health were open to the public and were reported in the press. The National Library of Medicine, Henry Leber Coit MSS., 16 boxes and 6 volumes of ledgers, contain correspondence, drafts of articles and speeches, published matter, and other materials depicting the life and work of the "father of clean milk." The Rutgers University Library, Special Collections Department, Consumer's League of New Jersey MSS, 8 boxes, include minutes, correspondence, clippings, publications, and other materials relating to the activities of the league for reform of child labor laws, improvement of factory and retail store working conditions, and enactment of minimum and maximum wage and hour legislation during the years 1913-1955. The minutes of the Essex County Medical Society for the years 1816-1920 are housed in the society's Office of the Executive Secretary. A candid assessment of the Newark Board of Health can be found in Bureau of Municipal Research, N.Y., "A Survey of the Government, Finances and Administration of the City of Newark, N. J.," November 1, 1919, in the New Jersey Reference Division of the Newark Public Library.

Index

ABOUT THE AUTHOR

Stuart Galishoff received his B.A., M.A., and Ph.D. from New York University. He is assistant professor of history at Georgia State University. Professor Galishoff has written many articles for scholarly journals in social history. His special interests are urban history and the history of public health.